Physician Well-Being
During Sustained
CRISIS

Other books by The Coalition
for Physician Well-Being:

Transforming the Heart of Practice:
An Organizational and Personal Approach
to Physician Well-Being

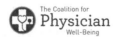

Physician Well-Being During Sustained CRISIS

Defusing Burnout, Building Resilience, Restoring Hope

EDITORS

TED HAMILTON, MD, MBA

DIANNE MCCALLISTER, MD, MBA

DEANNA SANTANA-CEBOLLERO, PHD

AdventHealth Press

AdventHealth

PHYSICIAN WELL-BEING DURING SUSTAINED CRISIS
Copyright © MMXXI Coalition for Physician Well-Being
Published by AdventHealth Press
605 Montgomery Road, Altamonte Springs, Florida 32714

EXTENDING *the* HEALING MINISTRY *of* CHRIST

Editor-in-Chief	Todd Chobotar
Managing Editor	Denise Rougeux-Putt
Internal Peer Reviewers	Jeffrey Kuhlman, MD
	Jessica Baird-Wertman, MHA
	Teresa Herbert, MD
	Eric Shadle, MD
External Peer Reviewers	Loice Swisher, MD
	Cindy Boskind, MD
	Roger Woodruff, MD
Copy Editor	Pam Nordberg
Promotion	Caryn McCleskey
Production	Lillian Boyd
Photography	Spencer Freeman
Cover Design	John Lucas
Interior Design	Kathy Curtis

For special orders, events, or other information, please contact:
AdventHealthPress.com | 407-200-8224

AdventHealth Press is a wholly owned entity of AdventHealth.
Library of Congress Control number: 2021911859
Printed in the United States of America.
PR 14 13 12 11 10 9 8 7 6 5 4 3 2 1
ISBN: 978-1-7372507-2-2 (Print)
ISBN: 978-1-7372507-3-9 (EBook)

For other life changing resources visit:
AdventHealthPress.com
CreationLife.com

CONTENTS

INTRODUCTION

Fatigue, isolation, worry, anxiety, depression, moral distress. We can't blame it all on COVID-19. After all, physicians were experiencing burnout long before the onslaught of this pandemic. The practice of medicine has never been easy—years of demanding education and training culminating in a career characterized by long hours; frequent night, weekend, and holiday call duty; stress-laden decisions and procedures; burgeoning bureaucracy and regulatory requirements; and now this—a worldwide health care crisis.

- How do we cope?
- How do we help our professional colleagues cope?
- How do we fulfill our clinical calling while maintaining personal health and stability?
- How do we adapt to abrupt and dramatic change in our practice patterns, professional relationships, and ways of carrying out our duties?
- How do we engage our associates, team members, patients, and families to understand and accommodate despite the barriers imposed by personal protective equipment, isolation care, unpredictable surges in demand, and unprecedented fatalities?
- How do we come back?
- How do we summon the energy to show up?
- How do we tap our spiritual resources for caring despite fatigue and prolonged stress?

The prologue to this book consists of the first-person experience of a physician who contracted COVID-19 and of the doctors who treated him during his illness. Those who ponder this story may well recognize signs and symptoms related to physician illness, stress, and burnout reflected among the professional participants as profiled in this brief narrative.

The book is a collection of essays organized around a unifying theme of well-being for physicians in crisis, with three subsections related, respectively, to resilience, organizational culture, and spiritual care. It is not a continuous narrative, nor is it intended to be read cover to cover, front to back. It is a practical resource, to be browsed as interested, consulted as needed, and applied as indicated. The observant reader will note some degree of repetition regarding the COVID-19 epidemic, its onset, course, and impact on health care providers, particularly physicians. We have chosen, in most cases, to retain the author's original wording, despite the repetition, since each one's experience is unique in various ways.

The first third of this book addresses physician well-being in a time of social and clinical crisis—in this time of pandemic. Contributors are seasoned professionals drawn from the frontlines of the COVID-19 battle. They are caregivers and those who care for the caregivers. They tell their stories and offer counsel based on real-life experience.

The second section provides perspective on the essential role of health care institutions in promoting physician wholeness. Research shows that physician resilience initiatives are more effective when individual physician efforts are augmented by organizational intentionality and support. Themes that surface in these essays include communication, collaboration, and trust, facilitated by organized, directed efforts to prepare physicians and provide support, not only in times of crisis, but as a part of organizational culture.

The third and final section is perhaps the most sensitive and personal in content and scope. Much has been written over recent years, in both scientific literature and popular press, about physician burnout and resilience, about the importance of addressing workplace inefficiency, about the need for personal time, rest, recuperation, and relationship with family and friends. But little has been written about restoring the bruised and broken spirit of a dedicated physician. These essays are about encouraging the doctor's heart, refreshing the doctor's spirit, and restoring the joy of practice.

The authors of this book include practicing physicians, health care administrators, chaplains, professional coaches, and counselors—all of whom are experienced and dedicated to caring for and supporting physicians. Our desire is that you will find, within these pages, encouragement, hope, and renewed commitment to caring for those who care for us.

Ted Hamilton, MD, MBA

PROLOGUE

Alan A. Nelson, MD

Dr. Alan Nelson, a practicing psychiatrist, shares his own experience as a COVID-19 patient and reflects on what went well and what could have gone better—much better. What role might the cardinal components of burnout—emotional exhaustion, depersonalization, reduced personal efficacy—have played in the process and interactions described in this story?

In many ways, 2020 seemed to be the year that everything changed. None of us really want to relive that year. The country was caught up in a pandemic, and medical guidelines were confusing and ever changing. America was torn by racial tension and political turmoil.

I'm a psychiatrist in solo practice. My spouse, Claudia, is a pediatrician with a primary care group. We both practice part time. We've been fortunate to have three adult children and six grandchildren. We have had a medical marriage for over 40 years and made it work.

We have lived though many changes in this medical life including moves, group changes, and periodic medical staff dramas. However, in 2020 we had a new experience—poor medical care and almost unbelievably deficient physician-patient communication.

We live in Redstone, Colorado, a small village at 7400-foot elevation in the Rocky Mountains. It's a beautiful rural setting, where the nearest hospital is about 45 minutes away. In the last four years, I've had to become acquainted with three new doctors since many rural physicians are limiting Medicare patients. Previously, I enjoyed a 15-year-long positive relationship with my internist, but he transitioned to concierge medicine. My choice of a physician was restricted to only those who could or would take me.

In late March of 2020, following several days of malaise and fatigue, late one night I just could not breathe. I've always enjoyed good health and had no history of underlying pulmonary problems. Claudia took me to the emergency department where I tested positive for COVID-19 and received care and oxygen for several hours. I had never felt so sick, but I was released from the emergency department and given a three-liter oxygen tank that would last me about five hours. They clearly did not want to admit me, and I refused to leave the hospital. I was eventually admitted, given good critical care (no ventilator thankfully), and was discharged to home four days later.

I isolated for several weeks in a cabin on our property. During that time, I received no contact from my doctor. Following three weeks of cabin isolation, I texted my new primary care physician and said I was feeling better, on oxygen, and thought that perhaps a follow-up EKG and chest X-ray would be helpful. I never heard back.

I repeatedly called the pulmonary center, as instructed, to make a follow-up virtual appointment. Multiple calls. Multiple days. No return call. I wondered if I should stop or change the medication, how long to be on oxygen, and whether I should anticipate pulmonary complications in the future.

If Claudia and I had not been physicians, we would not have known what to do. We came to realize that we would have to figure out each step of the recovery process for ourselves.

The internet and YouTube became our medical friends. After a month, the pulmonologist did finally call for a very brief phone visit. He was pleased with my progress and wanted to "show me off in a Grand Rounds." I suggested Hawaii as the location.

At my nine-month visit, I was seen by a pulmonary physician assistant who was kind but totally unfamiliar with my case. She asked if I had been very ill with COVID-19. I was taken aback and gave a one-word answer: "yes." She seemed surprised and asked if I had been hospitalized. I said, "Yes, right here at this hospital." It appeared that she had not read the chart at all prior to seeing me.

Three months after my final office visit in January 2021, I received a call from a pleasant staff medical assistant stating, "It's time for your labs." I thought, what labs? I thanked her for the call, but I wondered just what labs she had in mind. She wasn't sure. "Well, the tests were from some blood work that you had done." "And can you tell me when this blood work was done?" "Oh, looks like the blood work was from 2019"—a year and a half earlier!

I know, I know. We ALL make mistakes. We get busy and forget to return calls. All of us. We understand that. Amends can be made, and we move on. A more serious, and potentially deadly, concern occurs when neglect and poor patient care become "the norm."

I have always believed the best source of unbiased heath education for the community should be the local hospital, not the radio, social media, a podcast, or YouTube. Good information leads to appropriate care. We have all learned that irrational fear and anxiety run high in a pandemic.

Many times in the past year, I've been tempted to give up hope that I could have any significant impact on neglect in the delivery of health care. Let's be realistic, I am in a solo outpatient practice of psychiatry, living in rural Colorado. Many of my administrative health care contacts have retired or aged out. Many medical centers are struggling to survive. Talking about hope seems like fluff.

Hope is not a Pollyanna term. Hope can have physical, psychological, and spiritual components. Hope doesn't mean you can cure everything. Hope is about working out a treatment plan incorporating the best technology, communication, and comfort. Hope begins with good communication, and change starts with us—how we live, how we work, how we run our practice, how we train our staff. Our spirit and attitude directly affect the culture of our practice and the quality of our care.

In this era where many physicians are now employees of the hospital, these topics of health care, hospitals, and hope are directly connected. We don't just treat disorders. We treat the humans who have these disorders. We can focus more on compassion, communication, and the inspiration of hope.

It is my hope, and I love that word, that this book would inspire one other person to put HOPE in the health care equation. We all have a unique sphere of influence, and one by one we can impact our culture. Don't give up. As I write this, it is late spring and a snowy day in the Rockies. I think I have a patient call or two that I need to return.

Editor's Note: Sometimes we get so caught up in the routine of clinical duties that we neglect to care for ourselves and those closest to us—our families, friends, and colleagues. Dr. Nelson's story poignantly illustrates the danger of becoming overwhelmed by daily responsibilities to the degree that we lose a sense of the importance of caring, communication, and compassion. The pages of this book constitute a call back to the basics—quality clinical care combined with personal empathy and genuine regard for the unique needs of each patient—especially when that patient is a colleague and friend.

PART I

DEFUSING BURNOUT

CARING FOR EACH OTHER AND FOR THE TEAM

Whatever the causes of physician burnout, and they are protean, the onset of a global crisis lays bare and magnifies the incidence and severity of signs and symptoms experienced by caregivers who are directly impacted by almost overwhelming clinical demands. In addition to caring for our patients, our families, and ourselves, we must also care for each other, as difficult as that may seem. We learn that highly functioning teams ameliorate the overall burden and stress. Physicians, nurses, chaplains, professional coaches, and counselors provide helpful advice on how to support each other while providing quality patient care.

CHAPTER 1

FOR SUCH A TIME AS THIS: LEARNINGS FROM CRISIS

Omayra Mansfield, MD, MHA, FACEP

Introduction

The year 2020 started off like any other and held great promise. To mark the milestone of this new decade, many were even advocating for Barbara Walters, longtime co-host of the show *20/20*, to be the one who officially welcomed the new year with her timeless opening, "This is *20/20*." Unbeknownst to most of the world was that while we were celebrating the upcoming year on December 31, 2019, the first reports of a pneumonia cluster in Wuhan, China, appeared online, and the Wuhan Municipal Health Commission had issued a public notice and started examining an outbreak.[1] The following day, January 1, 2020, the Huanan South China Seafood Market was closed.[2] By January 5, 2020, officials announced that common causes of pneumonia-like influenza, SARS-CoV and MERS-CoV, had been excluded as the nidus of this disease cluster.[3] Eight days into this new year, the Chinese Center for Disease Control and Prevention announced that a novel coronavirus had been isolated from a Wuhan pneumonia patient.[4] This was the tipping point for what the world would soon know as the 2019 novel coronavirus, or COVID-19.

The Pandemic

Over the course of the next several months, we witnessed the resilience and resolve of health care and the development of a global pandemic. With this being a novel virus, the medical community was learning about the illness in real time as it cared for a growing number of complex patients. Information was everywhere, which resulted in a dynamically evolving approach to managing the illness and mitigating the spread of further disease. The wide breadth of rapidly changing information also meant much of it was outdated misinformation. In a statement published on January 12, 2020, the World Health Organization initially stated that there was no evidence of human-to-human transmission, no cases had been reported outside of Wuhan City, and health care workers were not at risk when caring for patients with COVID-19.[5] The next day the Thailand Ministry of Public Health confirmed that a traveler from Wuhan had tested positive for the virus.[6] We soon learned that human-to-human transmission was possible[7] but still did not fully understand how contagious a person may be. These were early examples of how quickly information would change during the course of this pandemic.

Initially the hope was that the virus could be contained and that spread to the United States and other countries could be avoided, but this proved not to be the case. On February 26, 2020, the Centers for Disease control identified the first case in the United States of community-acquired COVID-19.[8] At that time, 121 health care workers were exposed after caring for a COVID-19 patient, three of which tested positive. All three health care workers had unprotected contact with the patient. The sense of security in health care slowly eroded as the realization that improved personal protective equipment was critical to our ability to care for these patients. The conversation around personal protective equipment as well as utilization of possible therapies became the mainstay of our national discourse over the next several weeks and months as the United States came to terms with the first surge of infections.

The U.S. Food and Drug Administration announced on March 30, 2020, that it had issued an emergency-use authorization for hydroxychloroquine and chloroquine phosphate products, two therapies that could potentially help patients with this illness (but months later would be found to not have benefit).[9] It also outlined guidance to expand the availability and capability of sterilizers, disinfectant devices, and air purifiers. At this time, health care institutions faced the possibility of shortages of personal protective equipment and scrambled to expand guidelines on appropriate use. Many states grappled with asking citizens to quarantine or shelter in place. Whereas before the lay public may not have been familiar with types of medical grade masks, quality of air purifiers, and the distinction between airborne particles versus droplet spread of illness, these topics made headlines as we faced continued increase of cases in the United States.

By early May 2020, the number of confirmed cases in the United States neared one million and continued to rise and would surpass eight million by mid-October.[10] Portions of the country, including New York and New Jersey, saw increasingly critical patients who overwhelmed their medical infrastructure. Medical and nursing staff at hospitals faced caring for patients without truly understanding the nature of the illness, knowing its level of infectivity, or having clearly outlined therapies. While many grappled with managing this first surge, a growing concern arose around a second wave of patients that would develop as a result of the mental health impact of the pandemic.

Mental Health in the Second Wave

At baseline, mental illness is prevalent in our population and is often undiagnosed and left untreated. One in five Americans experiences mental illness, and at least 8.4 million Americans provide care to a person with emotional or mental illness.[11] Depression and anxiety cost the global economy an estimated one trillion dollars each year in lost productivity.[11] COVID-19 exacerbated an already present global mental health crisis. In a survey of 2,700 people from the United States, France, Germany, Singapore, Australia, and New Zealand, 67 percent reported higher levels of stress since the outbreak of COVID-19, while 57 percent stated that they had greater anxiety, and 54 percent said they were more emotionally exhausted. Half of participants felt sadness day to day and felt more irritable, and 42 percent reported that their overall mental health had declined.[12]

The mental health impact in the United States paralleled that seen in other countries. A poll in late March showed that 22 percent of Americans reported that their mental health had gotten worse during the pandemic, and that increased to 35 percent only one week later.[13] An article published in *The Lancet* in March also noted expected psychological effects as a result of quarantine that included post-traumatic stress disorder, confusion, and increased anger.[14] A myriad of factors contributed to and impacted the mental health of individuals and of the community during the pandemic. These included financial insecurity, uncertainty of the future, rising unemployment rates, social anxiety, and fear of a second surge in infection rates.

Similar to the general public, the teams of medical professionals on the front lines of the pandemic are also at risk of adverse mental health effects. A study published in the *Journal of the American Medical Association* surveyed more than 1,250 health care workers in China who worked in hospitals with COVID-19 patients. Nurses, frontline workers, women, and those working in Wuhan—the epicenter of the outbreak in China—reported the most severe symptoms. A significant proportion reported symptoms that included depression, anxiety, and insomnia, and over 70 percent reported distress.[15]

Adding to the challenge in the medical profession was that, prior to COVID-19, burnout was already prevalent, with more than half of all health care workers in 2019 reporting symptoms. Suicide rates among physicians were high, with on average one physician dying by suicide in the United States each day.[16] This risk was emphasized in late April when a New York physician, Dr. Lorna Breen, committed suicide after treating patients with coronavirus and contracting the illness herself.[17] Losing a physician on the front lines of the pandemic felt like losing a soldier in battle. Many in health care came to grips with the reality that we were at war against COVID-19.

Leading in Crisis

Early in the pandemic, many drew parallels comparing soldiers at battle to medical teams in dire hospital settings. Like soldiers donning gear for a hard fight against an enemy, so were physicians and nurses as they donned their personal protective equipment including masks, goggles, gowns, and gloves to protect against the virus. While soldiers in many cases are faced with uncertainty and worry as they may leave their loved ones to go to battle, COVID-19 created an environment where no one, including the families of our medical teams, was safe or immune to contracting the illness. The virus was prevalent everywhere.

The COVID-19 pandemic required leaders to be innovative, thoughtful, authentic, and willing to adapt to change quickly and gracefully. Communication was critical, not only to keep the team informed but also to bolster morale. Consistent communication from a limited number of reputable sources allowed for clarity of information, given how quickly the health care landscape changed, and it helped team members not be overwhelmed with the volume of information available. Critical elements identified early in the communication cascade were to be present locally, engage with frontline teams, and round frequently. This consistent presence allowed leaders to check in with the teams and learn what was working, existing opportunities, and ultimately what was most important and pressing. The rounds allowed us to gain perspective on the resilience of our teams and the opportunity we had to help strengthen that resilience. Frequent rounding also highlighted the need to have strategies in place to help our teams when they needed more mental health support.

Most of our teams are generally resilient and can recover from difficulty and stress with embedded positive coping mechanisms. Resilience is defined as "the capacity to recover quickly from difficulties; toughness."[18] Resilient individuals can endure repetitive stress, trauma, and injury and are able to bounce back. But even the most resilient will eventually reach a threshold whereby they cannot recover without adequate support and additional coping mechanisms. As stress levels rise, individuals are at great risk for mental health disorders and ultimately may encounter a time of personal crisis.

To manage the expectation that our teams' stress levels would be pushed to the limit, we established a structure to promote the resilience of the frontline teams while also creating a process to ensure easy access to additional mental health resources. We deployed frontline tools and trained our chaplains on crisis response, increasing their rounding frequency and sharing leadership strategies. As stress levels rose, quickly identifying mental health disorders in our team members was critical so we could appropriately triage and refer them to the right level of care such as psychology resources, mental health counselors, or social work. We prepared to care for people in times of crisis without delay and arranged to obtain psychiatric intervention and care.

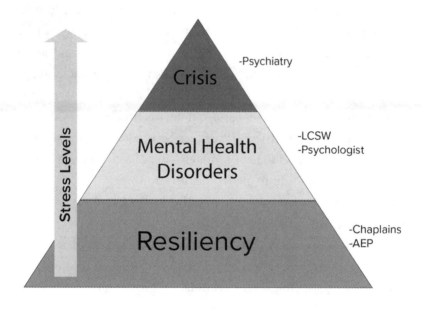

Adapted from Dr. David Buxton

Frontline Tools

Highlighting the similarities between soldiers and medical professionals allowed for the opportunity to learn lessons from battle and to share these teachings in real time with our frontline teams. In the military, a battle buddy is a partner assigned to a soldier who is expected to assist his or her partner both in and out of combat.[19] We encouraged our team members at all levels to identify their battle buddy for the pandemic. This person was a colleague who would check in on you and who you would be responsible for checking in on as well. This had to be someone you felt comfortable enough to be candid with, and vice versa.

We realized we would benefit from someone with an internal perspective of the current landscape who could tap us on the shoulder when they perceived we needed to step back from a situation.

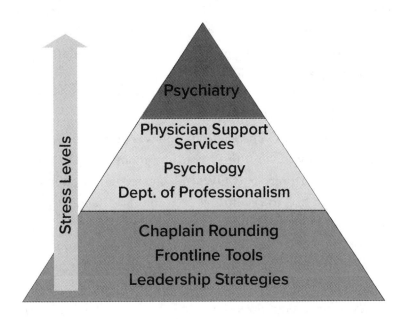

Adapted from Dr. David Buxton

At times we also benefitted from hearing the perspective of an objective team member. We leveraged the work of our chaplains, who provided an external perspective. Sometimes when we are in the thick of things, feeling as if wading through mud, our battle buddy may also need fresh insight. So we used the highly trained group of spiritual leaders within our organization. We deployed them to do more frequent touchpoints with our teams in a systematic manner and empowered them to tap a team member on the shoulder if they were concerned.

As individuals, we manage adversity and stress in various ways. During the pandemic, some used negative coping mechanisms such as excessive eating, consuming alcohol, and withdrawing socially. Many did not have a way to consistently exercise when gyms and other businesses closed, and many meetings became virtual. We regularly rounded with our teams to discuss positive coping mechanisms and shared behaviors and positive habits that we were personally using. We shared examples of positive coping methods that included mindfulness, self-soothing, and distraction techniques.

Leadership Strategies

Albert Einstein said, "The leader is one who, out of the clutter, brings simplicity . . . out of discord, harmony . . . and out of difficulty, opportunity."[20] COVID-19 created an environment where leaders had to rise to the occasion, lead fearlessly, and instill hope. Much of this work required being present. When much of the world was closed down, our medical teams were hard at work, and as leaders we were present alongside them. Being present and conducting frequent rounding with our teams had never been more important, and the insights gained were invaluable. During leadership rounding, we identified that teams needed a space to be able to get away from the patient care areas and decompress while at work. In response, we created the "Serenity Room," a space for anyone to use that had calming music, snacks and drinks, and a place to focus on the good in our lives with a gratitude board for team members to sign and comment on. Once filled with gratitude statements, these boards were then displayed around the hospital as reminders that good was still to be found.

Crisis is not new to our local communities. We have faced and recovered from natural disasters like major hurricanes and tornadoes, as well as man-made disasters such as mass shootings. These are episodic where the event unfolds and shortly after, recovery can begin. The pandemic created a challenge in its protracted course. It persisted for months with no end in sight. As a result, the team had to be prepared for a marathon, not a sprint. For long-term survival and to be effective, we had to be dogmatic about resting our teams and allowing them time to recover physically and emotionally. We developed contingency plans to account for anticipated times when leaders and frontline workers would need to step away for their emotional well-being and possibly even to recover from the virus.

Another challenge resulting from the protracted course of the pandemic was having a traditional debrief process after the disaster. We had identified journaling as a positive coping mechanism and encouraged our leaders to journal as a strategy to handle the stress of the pandemic. Equally important, we asked our leaders to journal as a way to capture lessons learned, scribing things that went well, as well as opportunities. This strategy ultimately allowed the team to debrief incrementally after the first wave of patients. At the time, we had no way of knowing that the following week we would see a second, much greater wave of patients.

Finding Joy in Crisis

Throughout this journey, we have been challenged with finding ways to safely care for our patients and to show compassion to our team. Very few outside the walls of the hospital can understand the stress so many health professionals encountered early in the pandemic as, together, we made our way to work each day on this journey of learning, uncertainty, and fear. We encouraged mechanisms for strengthening our resilience, modeled positive coping behaviors as leaders, encouraged open dialogue and transparency as questions arose, and brought in additional support and mental health resources. Of all these, two strategies in particular stood out as most meaningful to our teams—finding moments of joy and sharing "My COVID-19 Story."

It may seem ironic to ask people to talk about joy in the middle of a global pandemic. Yet sometimes, being intentional in seeking joy can help you get from one day to the next. We encouraged people to find those moments of joy so that when they reflected on this period of time at some point in the future, they had something positive to hold onto. And if they could not find a moment of joy, we encouraged them to create it themselves! I personally felt despair one day driving home after a particularly difficult day at the hospital. I had learned about predictions of what was yet to come, and the information was overwhelming. As I got closer to home, I decided to focus on creating a moment of joy as a way to counter the sense of despair. Upon arriving home, I surprised my two young children and husband by going to our backyard and jumping into our pool still in my work clothes, much to the kids' delight. The laughter that filled the air was a reminder that there was still joy to be found.

As the summer played out and we cared for an increasing number of COVID-19 patients, our team members were writing their own personal COVID-19 stories. Every person was impacted by this pandemic differently, and we identified the beneficial idea to create a forum for sharing stories in a space with other health care providers who could uniquely understand the journey. Initially "My COVID-19 Story" became a forum where our physicians could share their experience, both personal and professional, in a safe, confidential space with other physicians. In these conversations, we heard stories of what it was like to care for your first COVID-19 patient, what it was like to have COVID-19 yourself, or even how difficult the in vitro fertilization journey could be during COVID-19 and stay-at-home orders. The stories shared created a sense of validation for others who had been through similar experiences. These proved to be valuable sessions, and we ultimately started including the rest of the clinical team, with similar results.

Conclusion

At the time of this writing, we are still in the COVID-19 global pandemic. No vaccine is available yet, and we continue to care for critically ill patients. Our teams are now also caring for the large number of patients who delayed care during the pandemic for a variety of reasons, including fear and financial instability. Despite this, we do not despair. We have demonstrated to our patients, community, clinical team, and most importantly ourselves that we are resilient. We are stronger, not in spite of our journey, but because of it. As an emergency medicine physician, I am reminded on a regular basis that we have no idea how much time God will allow us on this earth. As such, we must live with intentionality as if each day were our last. We must find our moments of joy. If we can't find them, then we create them!

Omayra Mansfield, MD, MHA, FACEP
Vice President and Chief Medical Officer
AdventHealth Apopka and AdventHealth Winter Garden

Endnotes

1. Shih G, Rauhala E, Sun LH. Early Missteps and State Secrecy in China Probably Allowed the Coronavirus to Spread Farther and Faster. *The Washington Post.* 2020. https://www.washingtonpost.com/world/2020/02/01/early-missteps-state-secrecy-china-likely-allowed-coronavirus-spread-farther-faster/. Published February 1, 2020. Accessed 2020-10-13.

2. Huang K. Undiagnosed Pneumonia - China (HUBEI) (01): Wildlife Sales, Market Closed, Request for Information. ProMED. https://promedmail.org/promed-post/?id=6866757. Published 2020. Accessed 2020-10-13.

3. WHO. Pneumonia of Unknown Cause - China. World Health Organization. https://www.who.int/csr/don/05-january-2020-pneumonia-of-unknown-cause-china/en/. Published 2020. Accessed 2020-10-13.

4. Tu W, Tang H, Chen F, et al. Notes from the Field: Epidemic Update and Risk Assessment of 2019 Novel Coronavirus - China, January 28, 2020. *China CDC Weekly.* 2020;2(6):83-86. http://weekly.chinacdc.cn/en/article/id/24bdcf95-add0-49f0-8ae5-50abff657593. Accessed 2020-10-13.

5. WHO. Novel Coronavirus - China. World Health Organization. https://www.who.int/csr/don/12-january-2020-novel-coronavirus-china/en/. Published 2020. Accessed 2020-10-13.

6. WHO. Novel Coronavirus - Thailand (ex-China). World Health Organization. https://www.who.int/csr/don/14-january-2020-novel-coronavirus-thailand/en/. Published 2020. Accessed 2020-10-13.

7. CDC. CDC Confirms Person-to-Person Spread of New Coronavirus in the United States. https://www.cdc.gov/media/releases/2020/p0130-coronavirus-spread.html. Published 2020. Accessed 2020-10-13.

8. CDC. CDC Confirms Possible Instance of Community Spread of COVID-19 in US. https://www.cdc.gov/media/releases/2020/s0226-Covid-19-spread.html. Published 2020. Accessed 2020-10-13.

9. USFDA. Coronavirus (COVID-19) Update: Daily Roundup March 30, 2020. https://www.fda.gov/news-events/press-announcements/coronavirus-covid-19-update-daily-roundup-march-30-2020. Published 2020. Accessed 2020-10-13.

10. Worldometer. Coronavirus Cases United States. https://www.worldometers.info/coronavirus/country/us/. Published 2020. Accessed 2020-10-13.

11. Mental Health By the Numbers National Alliance on Mental Illness. https://www.nami.org/mhstats. Published 2020. Accessed 2020-10-13.

12. Qualtrics. The Other COVID-19 Crisis: Mental Health. In: www.Qualtrics.com/blog/confronting-mental-health; 2020.

13. Axios. The Coronavirus' Toll on our Mental and Emotional Health. https://www.axios.com/coronavirus-mental-health-coping-social-distancing-bf6fc053-4451-48df-9a37-0acb52c47e8a.html. Published 2020. Accessed 2020-10-13.

14. Brooks S, Webster R, Smith L, et al. The Psychological Impact of Quarantine and How to Reduce It: Rapid Review of the Evidence. *The Lancet (London, England)*. 2020;395(10227):912-920.

15. Lai J, Ma S, Wang Y, et al. Factors Associated With Mental Health Outcomes Among Health Care Workers Exposed to Coronavirus Disease 2019. *JAMA Network Open*. 2020;3(3):e203976.

16. Batista SM. Physician Suicide is Not a Passing COVID-Era Problem. *Psychology Today*. 2020. https://www.psychologytoday.com/us/blog/shame-no-more/202009/physician-suicide-is-not-passing-covid-era-problem. Accessed 2020-10-13.

17. Hauck G. 'Brave, Compassionate and Dedicated': ER Doctor Who Treated Coronavirus Patients Dies by Suicide. *USA Today*. 2020. https://www.usatoday.com/story/news/nation/2020/04/28/new-york-coronavirus-emergency-room-doctor-lorna-breen-dies-suicide/3038704001/. Published April 28, 2020. Accessed 2020-10-13.

18. Bing.com. Resilience Definition. https://www.bing.com/search?q=resilience+definition&form=BFBSPR&frb=1. Accessed 2020.

19. Wikipedia. Battle Buddy Definition. https://en.wikipedia.org/wiki/Battle_buddy. Accessed 2020.

20. Bodhipaksa. Albert Einstein: "The Leader is One Who, Out of the Clutter, Brings Simplicity ... Out of Discord, Harmony ... and Out of Difficulty, Opportunity." Wildmind.org. https://www.wildmind.org/blogs/quote-of-the-month/albert-einstein-three-rules-of-work. Published 2007. Accessed.

CHAPTER 2

WHO IS ON THE TEAM? AND WHY?

Ramona Reynolds, MDiv, MHA

Introduction

When a loved one is in the hospital with critical medical decisions being made, the decision-making process is chock full of strong emotions and long-standing personal and professional relational dynamics. In the midst of a novel disease pandemic, the emotional dynamics of care among the care team must be renegotiated, and the relationships between the clinical team, the patient, and the patient's family are realigned. This chapter introduces some of those changes and particularly highlights the shift in the role of the professional clinical chaplain in this setting. Using personal stories to understand the value of compassionate care and interprofessional relational collaboration, we explore how the necessity of the needs during the height of a pandemic may inform continuing comprehensive care for patients among the clinical team and chaplains, and the role of the chaplain in promoting resilience among the clinical care team.

Who Is on the Team?

"You didn't do everything you could do! If you knew what you were doing, my mother wouldn't have died!" "Maria" screams at the physician over the telephone as she hears the news that her mother has died from COVID-19 complications in the ICU. "I'm on my way there, and you are going to let me see my mother!"

Maria arrives in the hospital lobby full of anger and grief, determined to be with her mother after her death, as she wasn't allowed to be there physically before her death. Security personnel, who have stopped Maria from going to the clinical floors, call to see if someone can come and speak with this brokenhearted daughter. This daughter who has lost her mother, a once little girl who has lost the opportunity to share last words in the intimate way she has always related to her mother, is protesting the trauma this isolation has birthed. This now grown daughter has lost the opportunity to hold her mother's hand, kiss her forehead in her suffering, and peacefully say farewell.

As the care team arrives in the lobby, leaving behind the many other patients who are on a similar trajectory with this disease alongside those who are on another more confusing and difficult journey with the same disease, they are trying to steel themselves for the emotional attack that they know awaits them. The lead physician of the care team, along with the nursing leader and another nurse, invite the chaplain and join the security team downstairs.

As the clinical team approaches, the verbal attack begins. Seizing the moment when Maria takes a breath, the physician steps in front of the team and says, "I was with your mom; this nurse was holding her hand" and begins to describe how this team was standing alongside her mom in her final moments. "She was not alone." The physician affirms how this disease has taken too much from all of us and describes to Maria, who is a nurse, all that the team did in caring for her mother. She walks her through each step, answering every question. The attack ends, and the broken heart of a woman whose mother has died emerges. Amid all the tears, her anger transitions to understanding that they did all they could, they cared for her mother with competence and tenderness. Maria's anger turns to gratitude and an awareness of her extraordinary sadness for all that has been lost. Maria wraps herself around the doctor and weeps; the chaplain, nurses, and security officer surround the two in the sacred circle of loss to pray.

As the team is returning to the clinical unit, the physician, rinsed in a stranger's tears and thinking of her two young children at home, turns to the chaplain and says, "Pray I don't get the virus!" which reveals her own fears as she faces this pandemic. As the conversation with the chaplain continues, she says, "Being tough doesn't work with people in such pain; I have to be completely human." Being human sometimes means taking personal risk. More often, in the course of this pandemic, it means taking emotional risks and putting clinical care providers in places of vulnerability alongside vulnerable patients, as all of our human vulnerabilities have been exposed—physical, emotional, and spiritual. No one is immune from the exposure.

"Medicine is a team sport—the collective is often greater than the individual when it comes to patient care, innovative ideas, productivity and efficiencies."[1]

The team sport nature of providing medical care was never more apparent than during the crush of providing care during COVID-19, particularly in the early days when therapeutic treatments were more of a mystery and so little was known about the disease and the disease process. The traditional "team agreements" stretched in ways that challenged the individual's understanding of how decisions should be made and care delivered.

In this pandemic crisis, because of the isolation of families from patients, family and patient emotional support became part of clinical care. Nursing staff became emotional care providers on equal measure with their role as clinical care providers. Patient contact was limited, and the usual allied health team members, like chaplains and social workers, had less access to the patient; families were not present to provide support or to participate in care in the ways that might traditionally build a sense of comradery between clinical providers and family members. The distance only highlighted the disconnection, and in the midst of the unknown, the fear filled families with suspicion and anxiety.

Nurses—who are typically the connectors between the patient, family, and the clinical care team in communicating the care plan and timeline—are now adding to the clinical stories they carry: the patient's personal, human story. "Nurse Donna," after a particularly demanding shift caring for a man in his 50s, hears his life story, as he suspects he will not survive this disease and takes this time to do life review work, a common grief processing for someone facing the end of life. After hearing his story and overwhelmed with emotion, she shares with the assistant nurse manager and breaks down in tears. Her sharing becomes filled with questions that evolve to include whether she can continue to provide what she now experiences as dehumanizing clinical care, while feeling so emotionally connected to the patient and his story. While the family understands the need for isolation, even during the final days of their loved one's life, Nurse Donna is finding it difficult to face the existential questions of meaningfulness and meaninglessness, while at the same time providing complex clinical interventions. Her anxiety increases while holding this new role and simultaneously wondering if today is the day that she takes COVID-19 home to her family.

The clinical care team is more personally connected than ever before. The ever-present epidemic nature of this crisis complicates maintaining a professional emotional distance to allow for the professional objectivity that is such a hallmark of clinical competence. "The thin veil between the clinicians [us] and the patient [them] has fallen, and clinicians without adequate protection have become vulnerable victims of the same disease. The battleground is both pervasive and invisible; an airborne aggressor circulates freely among us. The possibility of death, potentially soon, has become the awareness of the new graduate nurse, the medical resident, and others barely beginning their careers and who now are facing the ultimate existential awareness of *this could be me.*"[2]

In the ICU, the team of clinical providers, led by the physician, might typically and most commonly include nursing, respiratory therapy, pharmacy, and a collection of physician specialists. In the United States, the experience of the COVID-19 pandemic revealed the need for additional team members as a part of the primary care team. Unique to this pandemic experience was the unknown nature of the disease and the individualized variations of its progression. This novel disease required isolation, which removed the typical emotional support available to participate in the care of patients. Clinical providers on the front lines of care took on the additional role of emotional and spiritual support for patients and families. This new role for the care team required new ways of coping and strategies for resilience in order to be able to continue to provide clinical and now direct emotional and spiritual care.

In nonpandemic "normal" circumstances, hospitals, particularly high-acuity areas like intensive care units, are fast-paced and stressful environments for patients, families, and staff. As "outsiders" to the clinical context, patients and families often feel quite disconnected. The pandemic heightened this experience, as the disconnection was more severe with patients isolated from all physical contact outside of their direct care providers.

Chaplains are resources for patients and families who need to process emotional and spiritual needs to connect their experience of illness to the rest of their lives. In the face of COVID-19, chaplains who have both theological education and studies in behavioral sciences, as well as clinical training, are really good at dealing with more than strictly spiritual or religious issues. They are trained to both address existential issues and provide meaningful support in the midst of a crisis. But the manner in which chaplains provided service during COVID-19 changed. While chaplains are often able to bring connection to the disconnected experience of being in the hospital, during the pandemic, chaplains were restricted to virtual visits with both patients and families. FaceTime, phone calls from outside the room, and other virtual communication tools took the place of sitting by the bedside and experiencing the patient with their illness or in the context of their gathered family. Besides the risk of contagion—which is an ever-present risk when working in the hospital—now heightened, many patients were on complicated and restrictive devices supporting their breathing, further disconnecting the patient from processing their humanity and making meaning of their story. The chaplain, often a bridge, now struggled in new and awkward ways to find connections to bridge.

Why?

Nurse managers and hospital administrators, during the crush of providing care for the infected patients of the pandemic, recognized an additional patient population emerging. Their own clinical teams were beginning to exhibit traumatic stress symptoms. As COVID-19 comes to your city or small town, the health care infrastructure and every institution within it changes. Now, almost a year into this pandemic (at the time of this writing), health care institutions are still changing. The need for emotional and spiritual support for the clinical team, as well as the need to support and encourage mental health conversations and resources for mental health care for clinical teams and the community, are just some of the changes that are needed.

As the emotional and spiritual support needs of the patients and families become more a part of the clinical team's practice, chaplains begin to see and hear more about the need for processing the clinical team's emerging emotional and spiritual needs. Chaplains become emotional buffers for the physicians and nursing teams. The intensity of the demand for care creates a crucible, changing the relationship many physicians have with their conscious awareness of individual finitude and mortality. Bad outcomes become more personal than usual, particularly in the early days, as the volume of bad outcomes overwhelms the physical and emotional capacity of the system and the care providers. "We have seen that spiritual care is not a luxury; it is a necessity for any system that claims to care for people—whether the people are in the bed or draped in protective gear."[2]

While patients and their families appreciate speaking to physicians, recognizing and utilizing the roles of additional team members, particularly nurses and spiritual care providers, is important. Nurses often have some of the closest and most sustained contact with the patient and family, and families often find consolation in speaking with the patient's bedside nurse. In the context of the pandemic, nurses are thrust into the role of spiritual care provider to the family. Nurses find themselves holding space for the family who can't be at the bedside. Chaplains provide care and support individually and in small groups for nurses, helping to shift the emotional load that nurses are now bearing.

Health care workers (HCW) caring for patients with contagious, life-threatening illnesses, such as COVID-19, are likely to have anxiety and fear of being infected. In the case of SARS, up to 50 percent of HCWs had acute psychological distress, burnout, and post-traumatic stress while caring for these patients. Fear of contagion and of infecting family members, social isolation, and additional stressors contributed to adverse outcomes. The stress of prolonged exposure to COVID-19 and the need to support clinicians have been noted in recent publications.[3] These statistics illustrate the emotional stressors that are becoming part of the clinical care team dealing with the COVID-19 pandemic, though foretold in past pandemics. As we look to learn from this experience, clearly the needs of the care team have changed in ways that must be addressed. Team agreements must be renegotiated. "All disciplines are ultimately responsible for ensuring that spiritual care is prioritized to improve quality of life and the experience of patients and families facing spiritual emergencies amid the complex life-and-death scenarios inherent to COVID-19."[2]

Conclusion

As all care team disciplines are making space for more spiritual and emotional care as a part of their care with patients and families, the clinical team must be expanded to include professional resources that assist those clinicians in finding spiritual and emotional support in the face of prolonged and complex emotional, existential stressors.

Acknowledgments

The author wishes to acknowledge Chaplain Edwin Alicea, PhD, for sharing his experience in providing care for clinical teams and families in the midst of the COVID-19 pandemic at AdventHealth Orlando. His experience and expertise informed and enriched the understanding offered in this chapter.

She further wishes to acknowledge the sacred stories of patients, families, and clinical care team members whose stories are shared, in composite, with pseudonyms to protect and respect their privacy.

Ramona Reynolds, MDiv, MHA
Chaplain and ACPE Certified Educator
AdventHealth Central Florida Division, South Region

Endnotes

1. Hambley PhD C. Five Strategies for Building a Better Medical Team. 2020. https://www.physicianspractice.com/view/five-strategies-building-better-medical-team. Published February 3, 2020.

2. Ferrell B, Handzo G, Picchi T, Puchalski C, Rosa W. The Urgency of Spiritual Care: COVID-19 and the Critical Need for Whole-Person Palliation. *Journal of Pain and Symptom Management.* 2020;60(3):e7-e11.

3. Wu A, Connors C, Everly G. COVID-19: Peer Support and Crisis Communication Strategies to Promote Institutional Resilience. *Annals of Internal Medicine.* 2020;172(12):822-823.

CHAPTER 3

ON BEING A WOMAN, A PHYSICIAN, A MOTHER

Jennifer Stanley, MD

One evening several years ago, once the dishes were cleared and put away, I was sitting at the kitchen table with my laptop, finishing up charts from that day's clinic visits. My daughter, who was probably six years old at the time, walked up to me, watched me for just a moment, and announced, "I am never going to be a doctor when I grow up!"

Taken aback, I replied, "But Maggie! I have the best job in the world! I love being a doctor!"

Maggie gave me a confused look and said, "All you do is type on that computer and act grouchy. I don't want to do that when I grow up."

I was speechless. How many times had I said essentially that same thing to myself? "I use my laptop more than my stethoscope. Who knew medicine would be more about records and clicking boxes and less about patient care?"

I know I am not alone in this challenging space—wanting so much to be an effective physician and more so wanting to be a good wife and mother. It is often a topic of discussion with other physicians and with other mothers. So often it feels one role has to take the back seat for the other to get ahead. Well-intentioned folks have advised me to "leave the doctoring at the office. Your family doesn't need to hear about it" or "You are so fortunate to have a stay-at-home husband. He can take care of the kids so you can work harder!" I know they mean this to be helpful, but thoughts like these for years drove me to divide and partition my inner self, as I tried to separate myself into "Dr. Stanley" and "mom"—which, I'll admit, was maddening. That evening, when Maggie reflected back to me that being a physician meant being tied to the computer, I realized I had some work to do. Not only did I want to show my daughter what my world as a physician really was, but I also needed to bring my mother and my physician identities back together.

I am a family physician in a small community and have been practicing there since 2001. For the longest time, I tried to be "just Jen" at school and church events, which was tricky. I tried to avoid engaging in medical conversations Sunday after Mass and after basketball games. I avoided eye contact with patients and family members at the grocery. Similarly, I tried to keep my family life private while at work, which became more difficult when my patients' children were going to school with my kids or when my patient was my husband's dental hygienist! Keeping the parts of my life separate was difficult, and honestly, I didn't do a very good job at keeping those roles in their own lanes. Trying to do so only contributed to my workload—and depleted my energy.

As a working mother, I often felt as though I didn't quite fit in with the other mothers at school functions or with the other women in community groups. I was often late to events, as I rarely got out of the office early. I usually brought something I picked up at the store, since I didn't have time to make any sort of dish from scratch. I couldn't join in half of the conversations around me. I didn't have time to watch the latest TV shows or to keep up on community events. I rarely was able to attend a daytime event at school—and when I did manage to, I felt like a novelty, as so many people remarked on my appearance.

As a physician who was not only a woman but also responsible for three young children, I often felt like I didn't quite fit in with the other physicians on my local medical staff, either. None of them had to make sure to get out of the office on time to pick up a child at day care; none of them had to cancel a day's office schedule to stay home with a febrile child; none of them seemed to have to ask for call trades as often as I did. I felt like I had to work a little harder than the male physicians in my group. The other women in my group were nurse practitioners, and I felt a need to differentiate myself from them, to prove that I, as a physician, was "more valuable." I picked up many extra shifts and calls while pregnant, knowing that my partners would have to cover for me while on maternity leave. I always said "yes" to seeing another patient regardless of how late in the day it was, wanting to prove to my partners (and to myself?) that I could carry as heavy a load as the male doctors.

Many of my fellow female physicians have shared these same sentiments with me. They too feel the need to work harder as physicians to prove that they are equals to their male partners, which often means stealing time away from their families. They have felt the same awkwardness as they try to join into other mom groups, which leads them to shy away from those gatherings. This only furthers the divide so many of us try to maintain between our physician and mother identities.

Once I gave myself permission to bring those two parts of me back together so both of those important roles could coexist again in the same space, I felt a tremendous relief.

To better allow my identity as a mother into my physician role, I now allow myself to talk a little more openly about my children and more often about my experience as a mother. I find that sharing little bits of my identity as a mother makes me a more effective physician. A patient reluctant to use a medication to alleviate anxiety and depression may be more likely to trial a medication when I mention that I took Zoloft for a six-month period to treat my postpartum depression. A patient reluctant to make significant changes to her food choices for weight loss may see an additional benefit to good food choices when I say, "I am highly motivated to make good food choices and try to model good lifestyle choices for my own children, so they will have healthy habits when they grow up." Pictures of my children line the walls of my exam rooms. Last Christmas, my oldest son performed for the residents of the local assisted living community, and several of my long-time patients were delighted to place the dulcimer-playing young man as the curly red-topped little boy from the photos in my office.

Sharing my experience as a mother when I serve as a physician peer mentor is helpful to my parent-physician colleagues. Having a shared experience allows my peers to recognize their own struggles in a safe space and allows them to explore their own opportunities for growth and resolution.

With the intention of allowing my children to see what my world as a physician looked like, I became more mindful about stories I shared at the dinner table or while riding in the car. I started to tell stories about patients whose lives I had helped, whether it was someone who had gotten his diabetes under control, someone who had stopped smoking, or a child who happily announced that she and her family now always eat dinner together at the table like her doctor wants them to! Sometimes I tell them stories that make them laugh, and sometimes I tell them stories that make them pause and think and then ask questions. We've had conversations about socioeconomic barriers, diversity, gender equality, death, life, lifestyle choices, and so much more. By sharing those real experiences with my children, they see through a window into the world around them. By sharing those real experiences with my children, I have the opportunity to reflect, explore, and grow myself as a physician and as a mother. I have also found my passion for medicine to be rekindled. Reliving these human experiences with my family keeps my focus on my work within the patient-physician relationship rather than on the distractors of charting, formulary limitations, and insurance authorization requests.

The stress of the COVID-19 pandemic has required me to revisit the journey I have taken over the past several years. As with any stressor, I am tired and have begun to doubt myself, feeling like my list of responsibilities has reached the length of impossibility. I feel like I haven't been a good enough physician—I was tucked away in my office seeing patients over a video, running meetings with my colleagues and staff over Zoom, rather than donning my personal protective equipment and walking into the emergency room to see patients who were febrile and coughing. I felt simultaneously that I wasn't a good enough mom—I was distracted by all the new workflows and communication my staff needed and didn't have time to help my daughter with her sixth-grade math homework she was trying to do online. I wasn't able to keep up with my high school son's assignments—and suddenly he was nearly failing chemistry. I wasn't a great wife—I couldn't remember the last time I had had a conversation with my husband that wasn't tainted with frustration and apologies.

A few months into the pandemic, a friend of mine asked that simple question, "How are you?" and before I knew it, I was telling her exactly how I was, which wasn't pretty! Weeks of bottling up the worry, self-doubt, frustration, and anxiety spilled out of me, and suddenly I saw myself through her eyes: a woman given simply too many things to do. Had I been on the listening end of that conversation, I would have thought, "Who does she think she is? Superwoman? No one can expect to manage all those responsibilities, much less manage them all well!" My friend let me spill my worries, and when I finished, she quietly sat with me and then gently spoke to me, affirming my state of perpetual overwhelmedness. She reminded me that Jesus, too, had a lot to do. He could have waved his arm over the masses and healed them all at once. Rather, Jesus sought out one person at a time. He made eye contact. He broke bread with them. He touched a hand. He spoke comforting words. He did God's work one person at a time. What a beautiful reminder for me! Why should I expect to do things differently? I needed to remember to take each responsibility one at a time, and in doing so, I have stepped away from those feelings of self-doubt and despair.

I have had to recall and bring back into daily practice those things I leaned on to better integrate my mother and physician identities. I've relied on my family (and our dog!) to hold me accountable to walk outside in the evenings, to take myself physically away from the unending list of work to do. I've relied on storytelling about how I, as a mother, have managed my own anxieties about my children going back to school in order to help patients find their own way to navigate the new way we do things. I've relied on storytelling to my family, telling about encouraging patient encounters in order to help me reconnect with the human side of my work, despite the lack of handshakes and use of my stethoscope during a virtual visit. When my daughter's principal asked my opinion on the school's reopening guidelines, I allowed myself to give feedback both as a physician and as a mother. I've given myself permission to turn off the computer at 6:00 p.m.—and turn my eyes to the dinner table, a game of Uno, or a walk at the park with my mom. I've also intentionally scheduled days away from the office so that I can rest mentally, physically, and emotionally. I am certainly not thankful for our current pandemic, but I am thankful that it redirected me to those practices I had already honed that foster and maintain my resilience.

When other female physicians ask me how I balance being a mom and a physician, I always respond that I don't seek balance—balance is static. I seek harmony. Harmony is alive! Sometimes the physician part plays more loudly. Sometimes the mom part plays more loudly. Sometimes it's all a little out of tune and I have to take a break to get it back into a pleasing sound again. I intentionally step back to *listen* to my world on a daily basis, in my morning prayer. This quiet time allows me to hear my world, and I can listen for things that may need to be tuned and for areas that may need to be silenced. I schedule my family duties on the same calendar I use for work—ensuring my family time is held just as securely as my work time. I have learned to discern the "spend" of my time wisely. I ask God what it is that He wants of me—trusting that if I follow His plan, I'll do the right thing.

Not long after the day Maggie painted my work as a physician as being chained to a laptop, I received a call about a patient recently referred to hospice care. I went to the nursing home to see her later that afternoon and took my daughter with me. Maggie, of course, was treated like a princess by the nursing staff, with cookies and coloring pages, while I visited with the patient and her family. On our drive home, Maggie asked me if I had "made my patient better."

I replied, "No, Maggie. I think my patient is going to go to heaven later this weekend."

Maggie was surprised and said, "I thought your job was to make people better!"

I explained to her that sometimes my job is to sit with patients as they near their death, to explain to family members what is happening so they aren't scared, and to sometimes give the patient medicine to help them rest or sleep so they don't hurt. I shared with her that often I couldn't stop the dying process and really didn't need to, that my role then was to accompany the patient and their family. She listened to what I said, and I could see her wheels turning in her mind as she tried to understand. She asked no more questions on our drive home.

The next morning, she came down to the kitchen and stopped by her goldfish tank. For the past week, "Silvey" had been looking sad, floating on her side, and moving only when Maggie tapped on the glass. This mother was ready for Silvey to go to heaven, as it was hard to watch my daughter worry so much about a goldfish! That morning, however, Maggie raised her finger to tap on the glass and then caught herself, putting her hand back down into her lap. She looked into the tank and then over at me. "Mom, I don't think I'm going to bother Silvey today. I think she's getting ready to go to heaven, and I'm going to sit with her a little while so she isn't scared. Is that okay?" I smiled at my daughter and told her I thought that was a good idea. I smiled to myself, knowing that my daughter had learned that important life lesson from her *physician mother*.

Jennifer Stanley, MD
Family Medicine
Ascension Medical Group Indiana

CHAPTER 4

WHO CARES FOR THE CAREGIVERS?

Bryant Adibe, MD

Introduction

I can feel my body beginning to break down: in the middle of a morning briefing, I'm nodding off; during an important discussion, I am forgetting the name of a long-known colleague. I am typically relatively calm, but as the days without sleep (and often food) stretch on, I find myself becoming increasingly short with my colleagues and others, the caffeine and adrenaline having long since lost their effect. It is day 20 in a row without a day off. On average, each of these days has been somewhere in the 16- to 18-hour range. Exhaustion isn't a strong enough word to describe how I feel. Nevertheless, we are facing a national crisis—or rather, an international, invisible war against a microbe—and in times of war, hours worked become irrelevant.

In our ICU, a critical-care physician berates me for what he feels is a lack of recognition from hospital leadership for all his hard work. In a quiet hallway, a nurse weeps softly as she confides in me about the emerging mental health issues her daughter faces at home. "My husband and I are at the end of the rope; we don't know what to do," she says between sniffles. "Can you help?" I can't escape seeing in her expressive eyes the worried look of a mother; maybe it's just a fleeting reflection of my own mom—also a nurse and single parent who carried the weight of raising four children alone.

"I am in constant pain following my injury. I've had three surgeries, implants, metal wires. I can barely stand, barely walk, and human resources recently informed me that I have exhausted all my available benefits. I need physical therapy and rehabilitation, and paying for these services out of pocket will bankrupt me. You came once and spoke to our department about the importance of well-being, so I am reaching out to you . . . hoping you can do something, anything . . . to help me."

"Had you done your job . . . he would have never committed suicide and would still be alive. You are a failure . . . you are nothing. We both know the color of your skin is the real reason you are in your role . . . let's be honest. You are a token." All the while, although I've told no one, somewhere in the back of my mind I know that my grandmother—the only grandparent I've truly known—is far away, in an intensive care unit, COVID-19 positive and battling for her life.

In 2018, I joined the Rush University System for Health in Chicago, Illinois, as system vice president and chief wellness officer. Leaving friends and family behind, I traded the California sunshine for the Chicago winters—enduring a brutal first winter storm that was among the worst in recent history (including a "polar vortex" with temperatures reaching as low as -50° F).

In Los Angeles, I had served as an associate professor and chief wellness officer for almost five years, among the first in the nation to hold such a title at an academic institution. I still recall how one of my earliest meetings took place on campus at UCLA, where I had the privilege of speaking with an administrator among those responsible for crafting their widely regarded wellness initiative.

"I am sorry to be the bearer of bad news," he began rather bluntly, "but you should find a new job."

I was taken aback. "Why is that?"

"The way I see it, this whole wellness thing will blow over. It's on the decline. In a few years, your position won't exist."

He was wrong.

Who Cares for the Caregiver?

The role of chief wellness officer (CWO) is a special one, particularly in health care. It is equal parts administrative and symbolic. Its symbolism is tied to a growing national consciousness regarding the importance of mental health and well-being—a consciousness further underscored by the psychological trauma that clinicians face during the COVID-19 pandemic.

As scenes of clinicians donning trash bags in place of adequate personal protective equipment (PPE) flooded the cable news circuits, along with self-recorded videos of nurses sobbing in their cars or providing tragic, behind-the-scenes footage from the front lines, a call to action was emerging. Finally, the public began to ask, "Who cares for the caregivers?"

Overnight, health care workers once regarded as pariahs—due to unfounded fears of their role in spreading the virus, at times facing threats or assaults when leaving the hospital—became heroes. From balconies in Siena, Italy, to grocery stores in London; down boulevards in Paris and from rooftops in Madrid; the world gathered to bang pots, wave flags, flash lights, and clap defiantly in support of the men and women who risked their lives caring for others in the midst of a global pandemic.

For some, the outward signs of support were therapeutic in and of themselves. After long days in isolation at home, they created a feeling of community and connection to a cause much larger than themselves. For health care workers, the signs of support did more than just lift spirits, they built unity toward a broader mission and created a sense of meaning and purpose.

And then it ended, as all parades, even with the best of intentions, must eventually end. But for the health care worker, the problems still remained. Many faced a lingering hangover caused by the cocktail of adrenaline, anxiety, burnout, and exhaustion. And to make matters worse, the pandemic was far from over.

The challenging issue of wellness in health care existed long before the COVID-19 crisis, just as the need for antibiotics predated the Second World War. But as history has shown us, it is often during times of crisis that innovation and significant shifts in our collective societal consciousness occur. These shifts led to the wartime discovery of penicillin during generations past, saving countless lives. Similarly, the COVID-19 pandemic can help lead a cultural shift in prioritizing the well-being of our caregivers.[1]

For years, threats to health care worker well-being have been well documented. We lose one physician every day in the United States to suicide. For first-year interns beginning their training as physicians, the average rate of depression goes up fivefold within their first six months of residency. This is also accompanied by a stepwise increase in suicidal thoughts.[2]

Nearly 40 percent of nurses will experience an extreme lack of empathy while caring for their patients, as a direct result of burnout.[3] Greater than 60 percent of pharmacists suffer from emotional exhaustion and other factors, also related to burnout.[4] These startling findings have led some to posit that depression and suicide should be considered occupational hazards of working in health care.

At the core of these issues is a flaw in our philosophy, a distorted prevailing belief in health care that more is better. By and large, hospitals are compensated by volume[5]—more patients, more procedures, more money. Departments are rewarded for meeting "productivity thresholds," which inevitably translates to being able to see and do more each year, often with fewer resources. Those who can keep up are rewarded with bonuses and promotions; those who can't are often let go.

So inculcated are we in this approach that we perpetuate and reinforce it, one to another. Physicians often speak with pride about their many sleepless nights, endless hours, and overwhelming schedules—all while bemoaning how "easy" the new generation of trainees has it, thanks to work-hour restrictions. Nurses who can withstand grueling 12-hour shifts are seen as strong and competent; those who can't are weak. The pharmacist who can take the most calls, handle the most challenging clinical patients, and stay the latest is seen as a *real* pharmacist, despite any personal losses or sacrifices incurred.

Sadly, this process of self-sacrifice begins long before these individuals see their first patients. It begins even before they're accepted into professional school and commence their training.

Anxiety, depression, and isolation come to define the years that should be the most jovial and carefree. The slightest imperfection in academic performance leads to an exaggerated response, a panic attack fueled by the feeling that their future depends on getting an A, in everything. By the time many begin medical school, residency, or any professional training, they have already experienced multiple rounds of burnout, and, to a varying degree, their tank is empty.

It's time to rethink the way we have been working.

The Case for Self-Care in Health Care

On the surface, the concept of self-care in health care should not be a provocative one. Ours is a field originally built on ideals like compassion, kindness, and healing. Somewhere along the way, we lost this.

In our rapid, unhalted march in medical breakthroughs over the past century, we lost the ancient art of healing. The pill has become the proxy for the warm touch, and the sterile procedure the replacement for the act of kindness toward others, as well as toward ourselves.

In some ways, we can blame our broader society. We live in an on-demand, always-on, convenience-driven period in our history, one in which effectiveness is measured in minutes, not in meaningful moments. Modern health care is merely a reflection of this larger cultural transition.

There was a time when clear boundaries around work existed: when the workday began and when it ended. People left work and spent time with their families or their friends. They recovered and mentally decompressed. But with the rise of the internet era and the resultant redefinition of a new kind of knowledge-based economy, these lines have become blurred.

With the same ease and convenience with which we can hail a car or have a meal delivered right from the palm of our hand, so too we are reachable at all hours and moments. On our way home, the emails pile up. At dinner, seemingly important notifications buzz and ping their way into our consciousness. And even though our phones or laptops may not be with us at the moment, psychologically, they are front and center. We cannot escape.

For physicians and all health care workers, there is an added burden. The same values that drive us into the field— empathy and a sense of duty to our patients—also keep us from maintaining the healthy boundaries that are good for us and for those in our care. Often, we end up placing family and personal recovery time on hold. Repeat this night after night, year after year, and like sandpaper, exhaustion erodes into our vitality one indecipherable stroke at a time.

So, when the prevailing belief system of an entire industry (also known as the culture) is driving its best and brightest to destruction, how do we change that? We start with ourselves.

Self-care is simple, but it is not easy. It is absolutely critical, but without effort it will be ignored by default. Once you have established a pattern of self-neglect, most likely during the earliest formative years of education and training, caring for yourself can feel counterintuitive, awkward, and even selfish. The truth is, without making the time to meaningfully fill up our own cup, eventually we will have nothing left to give—not to our patients, not to those we care about, and certainly not to ourselves. Far too many of us have been running on empty for too long.

Chronic exhaustion and burnout strip us of the very qualities that make us who we are. Our personality, creativity, and emotional capacity are the first to go. We become short with the people we love and increasingly insensitive and distant. Our bedside manner diminishes, and interactions with patients become more of a burden than a privilege.

Next to go are our dreams, the visions for our future that give us the fuel to rise above the day-to-day vicissitudes that can so easily weigh us down. The tragedy in burnout is that it makes us increasingly myopic, narrowing our perspective only to what is in front of us and in the immediate future. We are no longer moving toward an inspiring target; we are simply trying to survive.

Sadly, in its most severe form, burnout blinds us altogether, eliminating any sense of hope for the future or even for tomorrow. Accompanied by depression and possibly substance misuse, without intervention, this final stage ends in loss: loss of families, loss of relationships, loss of clinical privileges due to negative events at work, and most tragically, loss of life through suicide.

Most insidiously, we often have no insight to the fact that this process is even happening to us until months, years, or even decades have gone by—not until it becomes obvious that we have become a shell of our former selves.

Vignette: Kara

"Can you pass me that?"

I look up from my notes to see a young lady pointing at a stethoscope nearby. I have unknowingly taken her seat.

"Oh, I'm sorry . . . I'll move!" I start, beginning to collect my things.

"No need, I'm fine right here. I'm Kara, by the way." We shake hands, and I make a sad attempt at a joke. She laughs, though more out of pity than humor. She has brown hair, a slight build, and a warm smile. In the frenzied pace of the emergency department, her neatly pressed and impeccably clean white coat, along with her calm and slightly aloof demeanor seem out of place.

"Let me guess, you're from medicine?" I offer with a smirk. She laughs.

"Is it that obvious?"

"Yes."

"And let me guess . . . you are a medical student?" she responds. Ouch. Despite my best efforts to appear mature and experienced, she has just pulled my cards—a gentle nod to her seniority as a resident in the complex and archaic power hierarchy that's come to define clinical medicine.

We were in Palo Alto, California, an idyllic town just outside of San Francisco that is home to Stanford, and, more specifically, the Stanford Hospital where I was a visiting medical student.

My experience so far had been less than ideal. It was a beautiful and inspiring medical center with world-renowned faculty and exceptional training. But what it lacked, from my perspective, was warmth. A week earlier, on my first day, I had been rebuked openly by an attending physician for not knowing an important fact—all in front of a patient, who later spoke up in my defense. The attending subsequently half-apologized, seemingly more out of embarrassment than remorse. Reflecting back on that moment, I now sympathized with that physician, who no doubt was struggling with her own inner battles.

Although I would never have admitted it openly, I was counting down the days until I could leave Stanford. I had had too many experiences similar to my first day and had grown increasingly disillusioned with the image of the hospital where I hoped to spend the next several years in residency. I could never have known then, but my time there was a defining moment in my life—ultimately pushing me toward an unorthodox career path focused on wellness and hoping to rectify much of what I had observed.

My interaction with Kara was the polar opposite. She smiled and taught me things. She was patient, respectful, and made me feel like I belonged. Over the course of our shift together, I got to know more about her impressive background. In short, she was brilliant.

She had studied at Princeton and before medical school had taken time off to get a master's degree from Cambridge. She earned her MD at Yale and now was completing her residency in Internal Medicine at Stanford. Her pedigree and career prospects were nothing short of perfection.

Yet, in spite of it all, she was miserable.

"Bryant, I don't want to be here," she said bluntly behind tired eyes, looking up from her notes momentarily to take a deep breath. She sounded like someone who had finally confessed a deep, inner truth that lay hidden inside for too long.

"What? Why? I mean, your track record is amazing. What would you rather be doing?"

Her response was telling.

"I just want to be at home, with my daughter. She's six months old, and I rarely get to see her. All the education and training aside, I just want to be a mom. That's really all that matters to me."

"But you should do that . . . you can do that!" I said, stammering, half-attempting to give her hope and half-attempting to do the same for myself.

"You deserve that . . . if you aren't in control of your life, then who is?" I offered.

She paused for a moment to consider my words. And then with a slight knowing grin, as if to say, "you will soon learn for yourself," she responded, "I wish it were that simple, but in medicine, once you start, there's really no way to stop. You take care of yourself."

With that, she collected her notebook, folded her stethoscope neatly into her white coat pocket, and disappeared. Her shift was over, and I would never see her again.

Conclusion

By day 21 without a break, I had reached my limit. In the flurry of activity and adrenaline, I had ignored an important truth: when it comes to burnout, no one is immune.

I thought about my conversation with Kara, from all those years ago. I thought about those clinician voices ringing loud from the front lines. Finally, I thought about those long-standing, ever-present challenges: the colleague in desperate need of rehabilitation; the grieving families whose pain, while at times misdirected in its projection onto me, was a tragic reminder of all the work that still needed to be done.

In order to meaningfully contribute and continue this important work, I had to follow my own advice. I had to care for myself in order to care for others. This realization caused me to pause, re-center, and in the weeks that followed, it inspired me to make important changes that better supported my well-being.

Most importantly, I received encouraging news. Miraculously, my grandmother had been discharged. She was expected to make a full recovery.

If we want to transform the heart of practice, we have to start by finding the part of ourselves that we have lost. With the rapid, ever-increasing pace of modern life, we have unknowingly become victims of our own success. Burnout may be a complex and multifactorial problem, but on a basic level, its wide prevalence is simply a reminder that we have become unbalanced.

Medical breakthroughs in the past century have far outpaced any time in human history. We have introduced the use of genomics, robotics, and artificial intelligence, all with the promise of healing many of humankind's maladies.

Despite these many breakthroughs and the evolution of society more broadly, the core of what it means to be human remains unchanged. It is to this nature, and the inherent needs therein, that we must return. There is a beauty in this simplicity.

Bryant Adibe, MD
System Vice President and Chief Wellness Officer
Rush University System for Health, Chicago

Endnotes

1. Gaynes R. The Discovery of Penicillin—New Insights After More Than 75 Years of Clinical Use. *Emerging Infectious Diseases.* 2017;23(5):849-853.

2. Sen S, Kranzler HR, Krystal JH, et al. A Prospective Cohort Study Investigating Factors Associated with Depression during Medical Internship. *Archives of General Psychiatry.* 2010;67(6):557-565.

3. McHugh MD, Kutney-Lee A, Cimiotti JP, Sloane DM, Aiken LH. Nurses' Widespread Job Dissatisfaction, Burnout, And Frustration With Health Benefits Signal Problems For Patient Care. *Health Affairs.* 2011;30(2):202-210.

4. Jones GM, Roe NA, Louden L, Tubbs CR. Factors Associated With Burnout Among US Hospital Clinical Pharmacy Practitioners: Results of a Nationwide Pilot Survey. *Hospital Pharmacy.* 2017;52(11):742-751.

5. It is important to note that, increasingly, quality and even value are finally beginning to factor more heavily.

CHAPTER 5

PHYSICIANS AND COVID-19: DEBRIEFING A PERFECT STORM

Gregory K. Ellis, MDiv, BCC

Introduction

For some doctors, the fear of getting the virus is secondary to the pain of witnessing a degree of tragedy they have never seen in their lives. Dr. Cleavon Gilman is an emergency medicine resident in New York and was a medic during the Iraq War. "If you would have asked me this two weeks ago, I would have been like, *'Yeah, I'm compartmentalizing, I've done that through a lot of my life,'*" says Gilman, who says he grew up poor, in a working-class neighborhood in Lakewood, New Jersey, and lost his stepfather to addiction. Yet eventually, after weeks of ignoring the emotional toll, he broke down. He had to call someone and tell them that their mother had died. "After that, I just couldn't return back to the shift," he says. "I had to walk outside, and I was in the ambulance bay for like half an hour walking in the cold. I didn't have a jacket, but I didn't care. I was just crying, and tears just kept coming and I couldn't stop. And after that shift I just cried all the way home." ~ Anna Silman[1]

Such narratives are an all-too-familiar occurrence in today's health care environment. This would be true in what we might label "normal" times but is only heightened during a time of pandemic. A "perfect storm" rages, with clinicians operating in situations that threaten their own health and safety and that of their loved ones at home—with often limited supplies of personal protective equipment available to them—caring for patients whose breathtakingly rapid decline right in front of their eyes is unlike anything they have experienced before. And these patients, despite the best of medical care, are dying, often alone and bereft of what would typically be the family support so crucial in these moments. "It feels like that burden has been put on me to be like a family member to my patients," Gilman says. He used to put up a bit of a guard with patients. Now, he is getting them water and pillows, tucking them in like children.[1]

How can we find resiliency to meet such conditions and demands? When every day seems to bring multiple heart-wrenching circumstances, how can we maintain a sense of balance and purpose in our work?

Critical Incident

"The World Health Organization describes a critical incident as an event out of the range of normal experience—one which is sudden and unexpected, involves the perception of a threat to life and can include elements of physical and emotional loss. Often such events are sufficiently disturbing to overwhelm, or threaten to overwhelm, a person's coping capacity."[2] Such incidents can potentially result in very real consequences for clinicians, especially as they become cumulative in nature.

Physical Responses

Sleep difficulties; nightmares; nausea; headaches; diarrhea; muscle tension; agitation; increased blood pressure and heart rate.

Cognitive Responses

Poor concentration; impaired memory; difficulty focusing; intrusive thoughts; flashbacks; difficulty making decisions; second-guessing self; loss of a sense of control.

Emotional Responses

Anger; fear; irritability; sadness; grief; depression; numbness; anxiety; loss of trust; sense of loneliness.

Behavioral Responses

Self-destructive or careless; avoidance of reminders; change in appetite; increased use of alcohol or drugs; loss of interests; uncontrollable crying; argumentative; withdrawal from social network.[3]

Debriefing

In the mid-1970s, Jeffrey T. Mitchell, PhD, clinical professor of emergency health service at the University of Maryland, pioneered a process he called Critical Incident Stress Debriefing (CISD)—"a method of crisis intervention that addresses the sometimes overwhelming effects of a crisis, or critical incident, on first responders." CISD draws on the work of psychiatrists Thomas Salmon and Erich Lindemann, along with Gerald Caplan, among others. It is designed to provide initial "first-aid" for those who have experienced a critical incident and is not intended to be a substitute for psychotherapy. The CISD team usually consists of a trained facilitator, together with a peer of the group who has been impacted. "The goal of CISD is to manage the stress caused by a critical incident, to minimize further trauma, and to screen the members of the group for further evaluation and treatment. The entire process must happen within 24 to 72 hours and lasts one to three hours."[4]

The debriefing follows seven steps or stages:

1. **Introduction Phase**. The leaders explain the purpose and process of the meeting, introduce debriefers, and explain the guidelines for conduct (confidentiality, talk only for yourself).
2. **Fact Phase**. Each participant is invited to share his or her account of the event and his or her involvement in the event.
3. **Thought Phase**. Participants share their most prominent thought during the event.
4. **Reaction Phase**. At this point, the debriefing becomes somewhat less structured, and participants are invited to answer the following questions: "What was the worst thing about this situation for you? If you could erase one part of the situation, what part would you choose to erase? What aspects of the situation cause you the most pain?". . . This is described as the most emotional component of the debriefing and the one that allows for cathartic ventilation and emotional abreaction.
5. **Symptom Phase**. The group is moved away from the emotional material and into more cognitively oriented descriptions of current symptoms.
6. **Teaching Phase**. Symptoms are normalized and stress management strategies are reviewed.
7. **Reentry Phase**. The leaders answer questions, make summary statements, and provide referral information.[5]

Strengths and Limitations

More recently, continuing research has pointed to some of the limitations of the traditional approaches to crisis support, including the CISD model. Dr. Cheryl Regehr summarizes both the strengths and limitations of the Crisis Debriefing Model in her study on its use with workers in various emergency fields.

STRENGTHS OF THE CD MODEL	LIMITATIONS OF THE CD MODEL
Normalizing of symptoms	Inability to reduce symptoms of PTSD
Increasing control of symptoms through education regarding cognitive-behavioral strategies	Possibility of vicarious traumatization
Mobilizing of social supports within the organization	Limited opportunities to assess vulnerabilities of participants and risk of PTSD[5]

Table 1. Strengths and Limitations of the Crisis Debriefing Model

Response

In the face of the COVID-19 challenge, hospitals across the country are seeking fresh ways to support their team members' resiliency in the face of the unique demands of the COVID-19 crisis. "There's this feeling of being vulnerable at the same time you're exposed to all this stress—like you're rushing off to war but you've left your armor at home," adds Dr. Albert Wu, a colleague of Everly's at Johns Hopkins, and the founder of RISE (Resilience in Stressful Events), a peer support group for health care workers within the university's system. Wu says that this feeling of being under siege can result in panic attacks, depression, or anxiety. "If you are afraid or you feel threatened, it changes your neurobiology, and you are really much more prone to be in this sort of fight-or-flight response." Since the pandemic began, the RISE program has received more requests in any one day than they were previously receiving in an entire month.[1]

As part of our support for clinical staff on COVID-19 care units, AdventHealth chaplains established regular opportunities for debriefing and sharing. The goals of these sessions include:

- ⊙ Creating a safe environment and opportunity for all to share, or not to share, as they see fit
- ⊙ Providing active listening to the stories clinicians share
- ⊙ Identifying individuals (chaplains and others) who are readily available for individual sharing and reflection as desired
- ⊙ Providing education on coping strategies and signs of deeper stress for awareness (see resource below)
- ⊙ Encouraging caring for each other as colleagues and taking note of signs that others may need assistance

These sessions have been well attended and affirmed by our team members for their contribution to building resiliency. A by-product of this process has been that other units in addition to COVID-19-specific areas have now requested such regular sessions.

Following a group debriefing with a team who had experienced together the death of a young patient, clinicians commented:

- ⊙ "I needed this time to talk this out, because I just started thinking that maybe I couldn't do nursing anymore."
- ⊙ "It feels better knowing other people are feeling the same way I am, and we support each other."
- ⊙ "This session helped me breathe."

In another case, where a team was dealing with their feelings after multiple deaths in the same family unit, the group interaction allowed for the processing of their feelings about the immediate losses and also for sharing how COVID-19 was impacting their own families. This proved to be a sacred moment because team members were transparent with one other. A team leader reflected, "I am so sorry that I was not aware that you all were going through so much. I care so deeply for each one of you."

Resources are provided through these interactions for continuing care of self and others. On the following page is a resource along these lines:

Caring for Yourself in a Crisis

In challenging times, it's important to take care of yourself even as you take care of others. The following strategies can help you cope with mental and physical stress in a positive way.

Coping Strategies

- Focus on one step at a time.
- Acknowledge what you are feeling. Mixed feelings are normal in a high-stress period; feel free to recognize, acknowledge and name whatever you are feeling as normal. Grief is a significant feeling during stressful times – it is normal to feel sadness and anger as part of this process and at times, to be unable to hold back from expressing these. Own your feelings and allow yourself space to express them in a healthy way so as not to hurt yourself or others.
- Find someone who listens and is accepting. You don't need advice – you just need to be heard.
- Maintain a routine as much as possible.
- Allow yourself extra time to complete tasks. Be gentle and accepting of yourself and what you can do during times of crisis and stress. This will also help you be gentle and accepting of others in a similar situation.
- Take good care of your physical wellbeing.
  - Get enough sleep/rest.
  - Eat regularly and healthfully.
  - Do things that relax and nurture you even in less stressful times.
  - Some problems are beyond your control; know your limits and when you need to let go.
  - Escape for a time by reading a book, watching a movie or listening to music.

Signs You May Need to Speak with a Chaplain or Counselor

- Becoming withdrawn from family, friends and coworkers
- Finding yourself unwilling or unable to talk about what is disturbing you after several days
- Being preoccupied with a case or cases after several days
- Developing phobic fears about any out-of-the ordinary type event
- Having a disrupted sleep pattern (too much, too little, nightmares)
- Eating too much or too little
- Alcohol or drug abuse
- Reckless or self-destructive behavior
- Feeling isolated or without social support
- Being incapable of taking care of daily needs
- Feelings of worthlessness, hopelessness, or burdening guilt
- Thoughts of harming yourself

AdventHealth

Sometimes, a very simple tool can have a profound impact. The following checklist was developed by clinicians in one of our AdventHealth facilities and placed by the time clocks and other strategic locations as a reminder for staff to practice good self-care.

Going Home Checklist

- Recognize that you made a difference in the lives that you touched today. Not every interaction or task may have felt meaningful, but that doesn't mean you didn't make a difference.

- Thank yourself and your team for being the light in the darkness.

- Take some time to think about today.

- Consider one difficult thing that happened during your shift. Acknowledge that difficulty and let it go.

- Think about three things that went well.

- Check on your colleagues before you finish. Are they ok?

- Are you ok? Remember your team is here to support you. They will understand your challenges unlike anyone else since you are serving with each other.

- Now switch your attention to home, and rest and recharge.

AdventHealth

Conclusion

Supply chains have been stretched and challenged as health care organizations have scrambled to provide vital personal protective equipment for their staff members. Masks, gloves, gowns, face shields—these are some of the essential tools for fighting a pandemic. No less important are the emotional and spiritual tools to protect the clinician from collapse—empathic listening, readily available resources, the knowledge that one is not alone in the battle, the assurance that fellow team members care. Building our "stockpile" of such support will reap rich dividends through the resilience of our team members in their medical work.

Gregory K. Ellis, MDiv, BCC
Executive Director, Mission & Ministry
AdventHealth Central Florida Division, South Region

Endnotes

1. Silman A. Medical Worker's Looming Mental Health Crisis. NYmag.com. https://nymag.com/intelligencer/2020/04/medical-workers-looming-mental-health-crisis.html. Published 2020. Accessed.

2. Organization WH. Stress Management in Emergency Deployment: Health Action in Crisis. 2006. https://www.who.int/hac/techguidance/training/predeployment/Stress%20management%20in%20emergency%20development.pdf.

3. Counseling B. What is a Critical Incident? Bridgecounseling.net. https://www.bridgecounseling.net/critical-incidentefap. Accessed 10/15/2020.

4. Study.com. Critical Incident Stress Debriefing: Definition & History. 2017. https://study.com/academy/lesson/critical-incident-stress-debriefing-definition-history.html.

5. Regehr C. Crisis Debriefing Groups for Emergency Responders: Reviewing the Evidence. *Brief Treatment and Crisis Intervention*. 2001;1:87-100.

    See also Everly, G. Lating, J. & Mitchell, J. (2000) Innovations in Group Crisis Intervention: Critical Incident Stress Debriefing and Critical Incident Stress Management. In A. Roberts (Ed.), *Crisis Intervention Handbook: Assessment, Treatment and Research* (p.77-97). New York: Oxford University Press.

CHAPTER 6

GRIEF AND COVID-19: CAN HOPE AND HEALING COEXIST?

Juleun A. Johnson, DMin

"There is a sacredness in tears. They are not the mark of weakness, but of power. They speak more eloquently than ten thousand tongues. They are the messengers of overwhelming grief, of deep contrition, and of unspeakable love."   *~ Washington Irving*

Introduction

The year 2020 will be forever etched in the annals of time and history. The transition of old and new has moved at an infinite pace. In many ways, the normal rules of life as we knew before 2020 have been transitioned to living a socially distanced existence. In health care, opportunities to connect with staff, other team members, and families are precious moments. These normal in-person encounters have been replaced by a veil of extensive personal protective equipment (PPE). This new way of living using PPE has replaced the smile and warmth of an appropriate touch with a face mask, a gown, gloves, and an eye shield. In normal grief and end-of-life situations, persons are given opportunities to stand around the bedside of loved ones.

These sacred final moments are important for closure, religious ritual, and human connection with each other and with the family's perspective of who God is in that moment. Instead of in-person encounters, at times these final moments may be via a form of media: a phone, video conference, or other method.

This chapter is dedicated to assisting you as a medical professional, regardless of discipline, to consider the emotional toll on interpersonal relationships. In addition to evidence-based research, I'll share practical strategies to assist each person with experiencing ways of meaningful coping while serving in a health care setting.

Leadership and Reality

Between the Medical College Admission Test (MCAT), other placement exams, degrees, and retirement are a wealth of experiences, some too fond to forget and some too horrendous to remember. The global pandemic has caused a shift in view on the continuum of personal history. Life as we knew it has been adjusted. However, despite the challenges of a global pandemic, each person has been immersed into a new reality.

Tom Werner, former AdventHealth CEO, said, "The first role of the leader is to define reality. Without doing so, a person, group, or entity is on the path to repeat its most challenging days."[1] Avoiding the reality of COVID-19 and its impact on the professional environment is detrimental to positive functioning and productivity. As a senior executive leader, your team is looking to you not only for leadership but also for compassion. Opportunities for your executive team, vice presidents, directors, and managers to hear from you should not be given to other people. Your team is counting on you not only to be calm under pressure but to let them know you are fully present with them in the moment.

COVID-19 is a reality for every person on planet earth. No one can ever decide they will not be affected by how life has adjusted. COVID-19 has emerged as a term resident in the minds of many already-stressed physicians and providers. The literature is replete with examples of the core needs of physicians and how to effectively manage these critical moments. I would invite you to consider the personal toll this experience has invited. PPE shortages nationally have been a reality; questions are looming about the efficacy of one treatment over the other; and, finally, travel bans have restricted vacations and other moments of relief for every member of your team and organization. In addition, the new global vocabulary has been expanded to include words such as surge, flattening the curve, and quarantine. Each of these words can inherently contribute to a rise in stress levels and anxiety because they are repeated almost daily on many media outlets.

Complementary to the phrases are the feelings each person has experienced. I have been in countless offices of executives, leaders, directors, and team members who identify with the following emotional responses: "I feel isolated from family members and friends," "I feel lonely," "I am discouraged," and "I am smiling on the outside, but inside I am in deep emotional pain."

The most sobering reality is that despite the efforts of social distancing and emerging medical technology at the time of this writing, hundreds of thousands of people have died in the United States. The most sobering part is that the number increases daily at this point with no end in sight. But what about your grief? What about your pain? What about your loved ones? How do you process the continual list of people who are in need in your community?

The provider's reality is immense. While grief and pain are a true depiction of the experience of many providers, this is not new. In *Worldviews on Evidence-Based Nursing*, Jin Jun et al. quotes Di Donato Borgese in saying, "Each time a pandemic or an epidemic disease occurs, such as measles, scarlet fever, HIV / AIDS, Ebola or the flu of 2013, health care professionals are on the front lines, battling diseases and caring for sick and dying patients, even while knowingly putting themselves at risk."[2]

Since COVID-19 is new, there is stress with keeping up with the manifestations of the disease despite reading every day about the condition and seeing the disease up front. Protocols initiated to care for potential COVID-19 patients become obsolete tomorrow. Questions surrounding the efficacy of medication and treatment are a continual reality.

In addition to work, the providers' perspective on the pandemic is also apparent at home. Many providers are fearful of spreading the virus to vulnerable loved ones. One physician colleague shared with me, "Like other health care workers, there is a fear of contracting a virus that has unpredictable complications, from no symptoms to a severity that can even lead to death." Providers have been known to live in a separate room or in a separate state, sending children and loved ones to other relatives in order to keep them safe.

Everyone has a point where the emotional cup is empty. In the article "Clinician Mental Health and Well Being During Global Healthcare Crises," the authors cite, "Exhausted providers amid the COVID 19 pandemic feel the heavy burden of their professional duty to serve while running thin on personnel and making do with little rest and insufficient time for recovery."[2] In addition to clinicians, leaders have been running on empty. Some executives have said to me in confidence, "I am tired, but

I have to keep a good face on because everyone is dealing with something."

The thought that each of us can experience this pandemic without being affected is erroneous at best. Rachel Remen says, "The expectation that we can be immersed in suffering and loss daily and not be touched by it is as unrealistic as expecting to be able to walk through water without getting wet."[3] We all have friends who have experienced differing measures of the emotional weight of the pandemic. Instead of being discouraged, we have to acknowledge our humanity. At times, there is an expectation of the leader being superhuman. This is far from true. Every person experiences this pandemic in a different way.

Leadership and Self-Compassion

Real compassion begins with self-compassion. Everyone needs a person with whom they can debrief their emotions, troubles, and feelings. At times, instead of addressing core personal grief needs, challenges may arise. It is unrealistic to think that you are an impenetrable obstacle against hurt and pain. Instead of being able to express emotions with comfort, grace, and humility, anger may erupt toward the health care system, staff members, and our families. When emotions are depleted and grief is high, unnamed burnout may occur. Rachel Remen says, "We burn out not because we don't care but because we don't grieve."[3]

As a physician or advanced care provider, how do you grieve? Do you give yourself permission to grieve? Grieving in many contexts and communities is communal, sacred, and meaningful, so how do people grieve in a socially distant world? Many deaths of COVID-19 positive patients occur in the intensive care unit (ICU). In the article, "Complicated Grief After Death of a Relative in the Intensive Care Unit," the authors share, "In the context of COVID-19, bereaved family members may have limited support due to physical distancing requirements and may be forced to grieve alone."[4] These challenges of grieving alone are not isolated to the families. All health care personnel are affected by these losses. The wound of the losses is deeper than what it appears to be on first glance. In addition to physiological losses, other losses go beyond the walls of any health care institution. Loss of social and community networks, living alone, and loss of income are known to exacerbate psychological morbidity in bereavement.[4] COVID-19 has been translated to twenty-first-century leprosy.

To be sure, the effects of the pandemic are clear and present. But could there be unintended consequences of this pandemic? A sure and sound warning is given by the authors of the article, "Orthopaedic Surgical Selection and Inpatient Paradigms During the Coronavirus." The authors cite, "During SARS, health care workers involved in the epidemic showed over 90 percent anxiety or depression symptoms during the outbreak or after. Many had residual symptoms even after the disease had retreated."[5]

What if 90 percent of your employees or colleagues had prolonged residual symptoms of this disease? The symptoms, indicators, and factors surrounding cure of the disease as of this writing are still in clinical trial. However, the aftereffects of the disease to a large degree are still unknown. How does this situation affect the key relationships in your life? Ted Hamilton shares that there are relationships of high value and importance to physicians (in no particular order): patients, colleagues, spouses, and families.[6] How will you lead so that these relationships continue to flourish? One way for these relationships to flourish is by attending to your own needs.

Four feelings associated with long-term effects of care in an intense global epidemic are isolation, stigmatization, guilt, and helplessness, according to Massey et al.[5] The table below explores how each feeling may be experienced.

FEELING NAMED	DESCRIPTION
Isolation	Social distancing from family, friends, and colleagues after work Patients socially isolated
Stigmatization	Fear of patients having the disease Health care providers may downplay symptoms in an effort to continue to care for patients
Guilt	Balancing work and home life Risking exposing to self and family
Helplessness	Even those not involved can feel the psychological impact Leaders and physicians being seen as nonessential Concerns that a person is not as important as they truly are

Table 1

Building on the foundation of Massey et al., I would like to offer a perspective on how the four feelings and dimensions of challenge for employees and executives alike can be realized from a position of hope and support. Massey et al. share that isolation, stigmatization, guilt, and helplessness are core examples of stress during and after a crisis. I would like to invite you to consider four dimensions of hope during this same period. The four dimensions of hope are connection, identifying needs, empowerment, and freedom.[7]

DIMENSION OF HOPE	DESCRIPTION
Connection	Finding a group to connect with who can identify with your experience Having a battle buddy to help in coping
Identifying Needs	Creating some space to identify personal needs Owning self-care opportunities
Freedom	Accepting humanity Giving yourself grace
Empowerment	Controlling the things you can control Releasing those things out of your control

Table 2 illustrates the reality of the four dimensions of hope along with the description.

While these feelings and dimensions are not the sum total of resources for self-compassion, they are indicators to what may be useful for long-term resilience.

Leadership and Resilience

The final factor that helps the leader to cope and thrive in moments of difficulty is resilience. Resilience is defined by the *Merriam-Webster Dictionary* as an ability to recover from or adjust easily to misfortune or change. This is a stressful time. Your continual recovery during this time will be assisted by your opportunities to be resilient. In this final section, I will share some practical strategies for personal and professional resilience.

The following study may be something you may want to use for your own benefit in your location. Recently a study entitled, "Understanding and Addressing Sources of Anxiety Among Health Professionals During COVID-19" was conducted which asked three key questions. Eight listening sessions included groups of physicians, nurses, advanced practice clinicians, residents, and fellows (involving a total of 69 individuals) held during the first week of the COVID-19 pandemic, which explored three key concerns:[8]

1. What health care professionals were most concerned about
2. What messaging and behaviors they needed from their leaders
3. What other tangible sources of support they believed would be most helpful to them

The answers to the survey revealed core needs that each person faces.[8] ([1])

The answers were summarized into the following statements: hear me, protect me, prepare me, support me, care for me. I

([1]) Shanafelt et al. mention in their article that the eight areas include (1) access to appropriate personal protective equipment, (2) being exposed to COVID-19 at work and taking the infection home to their family, (3) not having rapid access to testing if they develop COVID-19 symptoms and concomitant fear of propagating infection at work, (4) uncertainty that their organization will support/take care of their personal and family needs if they develop infection, (5) access to child care during increased work hours and school closures, (6) support for other personal and family needs as work hours and demands increase (food, hydration, lodging, transportation), (7) being able to provide competent medical care if deployed to a new area (e.g., non-ICU nurses having to function as ICU nurses), (8) lack of access to up-to-date information and communication.

believe those elements are ways to show that each person, regardless of role, is important to the mission of the institution and community.

Sometimes those who provide care can be challenging recipients of care. Too often the desire to be in the moment eclipses feelings. But what happens after the rush of endorphins in a crisis dissipates? Each person is left to their own set of coping strategies. In the article "Grief During the COVID-19 Pandemic: Considerations for Palliative Care Providers," the authors share, "Health care clinicians are trained to put their own feelings aside for the patients and families. During a crisis this can be counterintuitive and problematic. Every caregiver needs a support system to be able to thrive, function well, and stay resilient."[9]

Resilience practiced and demonstrated sounds different for each person. At times, it's difficult to find the words to say to anyone. In my location, a team member I met in the hall shared that she had four loved ones die from COVID-19 in a period of three months. The losses occurred either out of state or in other countries, so she was not able to be physically present. What is a person to say when someone shares something like this? I have a phrase I use that assists me in my practice. The phrase is "I came to be with you." This phrase elicits support without a long-term commitment of time. Physicians and other health care executives are busy, but this phrase is a way to demonstrate meaningful care in a short amount of time.

I coach and confidentially support physicians and executive leaders on my campus and in my community. I have found that there are five essential qualities for thriving at this time. They are debriefing, fellowship, encouragement, support, and nurture. These elements take a different form with each team, but they are essential for connection and letting these people know I care for them.

Self-care may be the most valuable but underutilized tool for resilience. Wallace et al. share that during this time, self-care assumes many different forms. The authors suggest:

- ⦿ Find a time and space for grieving.
- ⦿ Make time to connect virtually with loved ones and friends.
- ⦿ Use self-care practices that energize you.
- ⦿ Seek professional confidential counseling.[9]

Another tool for support is journaling. Journaling provides a confidential outlet to assist you in processing your feelings and emotions without feeling judged or concerned about saying something right. Journaling is a time to chronicle your experience for future use, education, and inspiration. Your journaling could inspire wellness for the next generation of physicians.

There are four key questions and statements that I use to assist those I am coaching and supporting in my practice of care. These four elements offer an invitation to conversation as someone who is supportive. These questions are also useful for personal reflection to support and aid a person's growth. I have found that these statements assist persons in finding a window of hope through their grief. The four phases of grief recovery include:

- ⦿ Identifying the points of grief—who or what are you grieving?
- ⦿ Acknowledging the grief—embrace the grief, give it a hug, don't avoid it.
- ⦿ Grace—accept and claim your humanity.

⊙ Growth—give yourself permission to learn something new that benefits patients, staff, and yourself.

Conclusion

Finally, in order to see those around us and those we care for thrive during this pandemic, you must lead by example. Model and support resilience scheduling and activities. Encourage volunteer activities, encourage mourning, encourage meaning making, and encourage spiritual practices. Before you encourage others to participate in the venture of healing through these difficult moments the pandemic has to offer, make sure you take care of your own needs. You will be an example to the next generation of physicians as a result of this pandemic. I am so excited that the pandemic gives an opportunity for new rules to be written. My hope is that you write with a pen from a heart that transforms the practice of care for the next generation.

Juleun A. Johnson, DMin
Director, Mission & Ministry
AdventHealth Celebration

Endnotes

1. Werner T. AdventHealth Executive Leadership Program Forum. In:August 2019.

2. Jun J, Tucker S, Tucker S, Melnyk BM. Clinician Mental Health and Well-Being During Global Healthcare Crises: Evidence Learned From Prior Epidemics for COVID-19 Pandemic. *Worldviews on Evidence-Based Nursing.* 2020.

3. Remen RN. *Kitchen Table Wisdom: Stories That Heal.* New York: Riverhead Books; 2006.

4. Kentish-Barnes N, Chaize M, Seegers V, et al. Complicated Grief after Death of a Relative in the Intensive Care Unit. *European Respiratory Journal.* 2015;45(5):1341-1352.

5. Massey PA, McClary K, Zhang AS, Savoie FH, Barton RS. Orthopaedic Surgical Selection and Inpatient Paradigms During the Coronavirus (COVID-19) Pandemic. *Journal of the American Academy of Orthopaedic Surgeons.* 2020;28(11):436-450.

6. Hamilton T. A Single Step and a Thousand Miles. In: *Transforming the Heart of Practice.* Cham: Springer Nature; 2019:91-95.

7. Johnson JA. "Grief and Covid-19: Can Hope and Healing Coexist?" In *Coalition on Physician Well-being,* May 2020.

8. Shanafelt T, Ripp J, Trockel M. Understanding and Addressing Sources of Anxiety Among Health Care Professionals During the COVID-19 Pandemic. *JAMA.* 2020;323(21):2133-2134.

9. Wallace C, Wladkowski S, Gibson A, White P. Grief During the COVID-19 Pandemic: Considerations for Palliative Care Providers. *Journal of Pain and Symptom Management.* 2020;60(1):e70-e76.

CHAPTER 7

"I'VE NEVER TALKED ABOUT THIS BEFORE"

Liz Ferron, MSW, LICSW

"I've never talked about this before, and, frankly, it feels very freeing."

Some version of this proclamation is a frequent refrain from the hundreds of physicians I have spoken with, looking for help to improve their well-being.

Working as the physician practice lead for VITAL WorkLife, my role is that of triage for a well-being and support program for physicians and other clinicians—the program is purchased by health care organizations and offered to their clinicians as a benefit. I provide "in the moment" support, conduct well-being assessments, and guide callers looking for assistance to the most appropriate resource within our program, such as confidential coaching or counseling. I also attempt to normalize some of the difficult experiences and feelings callers express so they know they are not alone.

There is a cloak of secrecy and silence in medicine, and many physicians believe they are alone with job-related doubts, fears, frustrations, and sadness common to those practicing medicine. In fact, practicing medicine is considered one of the loneliest occupations.[1]

In an interview with Linda Schapira, MD, published by Medscape,[2] Tait Shanafelt, MD, noted the following, "As physicians, we generally don't reveal our vulnerabilities or the things we're struggling with to our colleagues. Many of these behaviors are reinforced as professional norms during training. Our training systems, even today, tend to be based on overwork and trial by fire and do not necessarily encourage vulnerability with colleagues." This is a real issue for physicians who often set unrealistically high standards for themselves and fall prey to overly harsh self-criticism and doubt unless held in check by colleagues and mentors.

I've found that normalizing clinician experiences is particularly important to those who may have shame around the reason for contact, i.e., failure to effectively manage their time, embarrassment about receiving negative feedback in their interactions with nurses, lack of marital support for their practice challenges, difficulty with emotional regulation, or fear of making a medical error. Most find it helpful to hear that I regularly talk with clinicians about these kinds of experiences, and their challenges are common in today's changing, complicated, and fast-paced environment.

Normalizing experiences and perceptions and helping clinicians to avoid being caught in unreasonable self-criticism can be important even to those dealing with everyday medical practice stressors. You may be familiar with the work of Glen Gabbard, MD, who first talked about the compulsivity triad many physicians possess, which consists of doubt, guilt feelings, and an exaggerated sense of responsibility.[3] Gabbard stated that this triad can lead to an inappropriate and excessive sense of responsibility for things beyond one's control as well as chronic feelings of "not doing enough." Left to their own devices, clinicians will often simply be too hard on themselves and carry the associated heaviness and difficult feelings.

Several years ago, I was presenting to a group of oncologists and posed the question, "Who do you have to talk with when experiencing the patient losses so common in your specialty?" I was surprised to hear that many responded with having NEVER had such conversations with colleagues. Times are changing, and medical schools now place far more emphasis on self-care and encourage future doctors to debrief after difficult situations with colleagues. But in day-to-day practice, time pressures, competition, and cultural norms still lead to "nose to the grindstone" and "grin and bear it" practices in response to challenging situations.

In addition to difficulties in speaking openly with colleagues about their challenges, clinicians face a number of barriers in seeking outside help and support. VITAL WorkLife conducted a 2017 national study on solutions for addressing stress and burnout. Over 60 percent of physician respondents reported six or more barriers to accessing well-being resources. The most common barriers were time and accessibility constraints and the stigma associated with seeking help.[4]

Another common barrier is the fear of needing to report having sought care at recredentialing or license renewal. Although efforts are now being made to remove questions about mental health from license renewals, the practice remains and is often cited as a significant barrier to clinicians seeking help.

VITAL WorkLife developed this unique physician well-being program, keeping in mind the need to remove common barriers for clinicians seeking support. We have been surprised at the high level of engagement of physicians and other clinicians—the same or higher than engagement in our well-being programs for nonclinicians in health care or other industries.

Our findings would suggest clinicians really do "want to talk about it," and we believe if they are able to do so sooner rather than later, the high rates of depression, chemical dependency, and suicide in this population could be reduced.

Regardless of whether clinicians seek avenues for emotional support more informally or through organized support resources, efforts need to be made by health care leaders to encourage this behavior and be part of the conversation to destigmatize the use of these resources.

What Can Organizations Do to Set the Conditions for Physicians to Be More Likely to Talk About Their Feelings and Experiences?

⊙ On-site support groups offer clinicians an easy access and effective opportunity to share their experiences with peers. Groups are often arranged by spiritual care, a well-being committee, a chief wellness officer, an employee assistance program, or through a more grassroots effort. Groups can be drop-in or available only to those who have preregistered. There are formal programs, such as Schwartz Rounds®, which offer health care providers a regularly scheduled time to openly and honestly discuss the social and emotional issues they face in caring for patients and families. Membership in The Schwartz Center is required to access resources for starting a Schwartz Rounds® program.

⊙ Encourage informal dialogues between peers by office sharing, offering a clinician lounge or coffee shop, time for interaction and "check-ins" built into staff meetings.

⊙ Create a culture of acceptance where fear does not abound, particularly in relation to medical errors.

⊙ Offer critical incident debriefings, which are often facilitated by representatives from an organization's spiritual care department or employee assistance program.

⊙ Arrange social gatherings and include spouses or partners, allowing clinicians to take time for socializing without compromising family time.

⊙ Offer internal and external resources for support. Accessibility, ensured confidentiality, endorsement by leaders, and a high level of promotion are important to success. Including a peer component, a virtual concierge, nondiagnostic counseling (such as what is offered through an EAP), and multiple points of access are important. Programs offered specifically for physicians or other clinicians seem to lead to greater engagement. Develop an internal or external peer coaching program. Our peer coaching program has demonstrated a 58 percent improvement in well-being scores from pre- to post-coaching. Physicians report three outcomes of coaching that have been most beneficial: improved confidence, improved self-awareness, and emotional validation.[5]

⊙ Establish internal well-being champions. Setting the conditions for clinicians to be open with their emotions and experiences cannot be the job of one or two people alone, particularly in today's large, often spread-out and compartmentalized health care systems. Champions reach out to colleagues informally and can sponsor various events focused on the promotion of well-being in medicine. Active and engaged well-being champions help keep the need for self-care and emotional support front and center.

Making Connections with Colleagues Independently

"I am not happy in my work," the young physician announced to me during a call. "I've been at this a year, and I still feel uncertain, overwhelmed, and like I'm simply 'not enough' during my clinic days." She went on to describe what is frequently referred to as the "imposter syndrome," where someone feels they are in a profession for which they are unqualified.

How could she test her perception of her abilities? How could she get meaningful feedback about her level of medical knowledge and skill retention? How could she find out if physicians like her were having similar perceptions of their abilities? To do so would require her to proactively break her isolation and speak openly with colleagues. But this was not an easy step for her to take.

Several studies have demonstrated improved well-being when physicians are brought together on a regular basis to share their professional experiences, feelings, reactions, and perceptions.[6,7] But what if this type of group is not readily available to clinicians? What can they do?

Simply put, clinicians need to be prepared to put effort into relationship building. It's hard work and needs to be intentional. But it has the potential to pay off significantly in terms of improved well-being, energy, and focus. When talking with clinicians, I recommend the following:

⊙ Identify one or two colleagues with whom you think you can connect. Ask one of them to go to coffee or, alternatively, a short walking break. Ask them how things are going for them at work—what do they find the most rewarding? Challenging? The goal is to build a connection with someone at work you can trust and can regularly talk with about rewards and challenges. Colleagues in similar situations will likely be able to understand in ways others cannot.

⊙ Get some of your colleagues together for a Zoom reunion or a socially distant social activity.

⊙ Join an online or virtual physician support group, such as https://www.facebook.com/physicianmomsgroup/ or https://www.pri.com/covid-19-group-support-virtual-meetings-for-physicians-medical-professionals-and-healthcare-workers

What Can an Individual Do to Support a Peer They Are Concerned About?

When someone is distressed, those closest to the person are often able to pick up cues from their behavior. Individuals in medicine often spend most of their waking hours in the workplace with constant demands and few opportunities to connect with their colleagues. When a clinician is feeling burned out or stressed or is struggling at home or work, often colleagues are the first to notice. Being sensitive to these situations can help clinicians play a critical role in helping their colleagues establish and maintain well-being and move toward healthier coping.

A distressed colleague may not ask for help, but that doesn't mean it isn't wanted or needed.

In discussing this issue with clinicians, I often advise the following: If you know a colleague who is distressed, it's common to feel unsure about what to do. If a colleague seems irritable or agitated, you may ask yourself, "Is my colleague just blowing off steam, or is there something truly wrong that requires help?"

You may notice that your colleague is withdrawing, isolating themselves, or acting in a way that is abnormal for them. You may wonder if it's a good idea to approach the person at all, and, if you do, you may be concerned about what you should say. Know there is no "right way" to handle these situations. The important thing is to reach out early and encourage your colleague to share what is going on and, if appropriate, to seek care. There are a lot of ways you can help a colleague when they have expressed a need for support. The following talking points may help to guide your conversation:

- In many cases, simply listening or validating the person's distress can be enough.
- Let your colleague know you are concerned and that they are valued.
- Focus on your colleague's strengths and, if appropriate, be prepared to offer professional resources for support.
- You may find the concerns they bring forward are NOT those you've experienced. Remember that everyone has different tolerance levels and different triggers, and avoid reacting in a dismissive or diminishing way.
- You are there for support, not to fix their concerns. Avoid clichés like, "I'm sure you'll manage," "Be strong," or "Everyone has problems." Avoid offering advice unless you are specifically asked to do so. "Fix it" strategies can shut down the conversation and leave your colleague feeling embarrassed about bringing up their concerns.
- Acknowledge the person's distress and ask what does make life worth living right now. He or she can create this list and use it as a reminder when feeling low.
- Identify the person's positive coping skills, and recall how he or she dealt with problems in the past.

Talking through feelings and experiences is an important way for clinicians to rebuild well-being and confidence.

Remember the young physician I referred to earlier struggling with imposter syndrome? "I couldn't believe what a relief it was to start to talk with some of my colleagues about what I was feeling," she noted after overcoming her reluctance to reach out to her peers. "It's made a huge difference to realize that others, even those with more experience, were having some of the same challenges as me."

She also found many of the approaches she was taking with her patients were the same as those of her peers, but noted when she asked for advice, she discovered strategies for making her job easier and more effective. "I'm definitely feeling more positive about my practice right now," she said, "and definitely not so alone."

Liz Ferron, MSW, LICSW
Physician Practice Lead
VITAL WorkLife

Endnotes

1. Shawn Achor GRK, Andrew Reece and Alexi Robichaux. America's Loneliest Workers, According to Research. *Harvard Business Review.* 2018.

2. Shanafelt T. Isolation and Burnout in Physician Culture: Innovative Solutions. In: Lidia Schapira M, ed. Medscape2018.

3. Gabbard GO. The role of compulsiveness in the normal physician. *JAMA: The Journal of the American Medical Association.* 1985;254(20):2926-2929.

4. Search VWaC. 2017 Physician & Advanced Practitioner Well Being Solutions Survey Report. https://info.vitalworklife.com/2017-survey-report. Published 2017. Accessed.

5. WorkLife V. Peer Coaching White Paper. https://info.vitalworklife.com/peer-coaching-white-paper-sign-up. Accessed.

6. West CP, Dyrbye LN, Rabatin JT, et al. Intervention to Promote Physician Well-being, Job Satisfaction, and Professionalism. 2014.

7. West CP, Dyrbye LN, Satele D, Shanafelt T. A randomized controlled trial evaluating the effect of COMPASS (Colleagues Meeting to Promote and Sustain Satisfaction) small group sessions on physician well-being, meaning, and job satisfaction. *Journal of General Internal Medicine.* 2015;30:S89.

CHAPTER 8

VIRTUAL CARE FOR CAREGIVERS

DeAnna Santana-Cebollero, PhD
Mary Wolf, MS, LPC-MH

Introduction

The impact of COVID-19 quickly reached the far ends of this world. This was not a pandemic specific to any particular country or continent, gender, or social class. The world started to shut down, country by country and within weeks.

Hospitals and health care systems began making space for additional beds, locating and ordering more personal protective equipment (PPE) and creating processes to determine how patients would be prioritized to receive a ventilator if the situation reached this point.

Clinical teams prepared for an influx of patients. Every day, there seemed to be a new symptom added to the already long list of symptoms.

The uncertainty demanded rapid response, daily learning, and enormous trust. Revise, redo, and refocus became the norm when it came to processes and procedures. Administrators and providers all felt the moral distress of questioning, "Are we doing the right thing, in the right order, and in the right time?"

To add to the challenge, many physicians began transitioning their clinical care from face-to-face visits into a virtual setting.

Redoing Events to a Virtual Platform at AdventHealth

Overnight, the programs we had created or redesigned to support our physicians and advanced practice providers (APPs) were set aside, and we had to adjust our plan. What could we do to support our team during a time like no one had ever experienced before?

My concerns stemmed from something Doug Wysockey-Johnson wrote in *Transforming the Heart of Practice*. He asked experienced doctors what advice they would offer to a graduating class. From that conversation, he states, "This group of experienced physicians offer the deep insight that relationships and collegiality are critical if one is to survive and thrive in the practice of medicine."[1]

With just a few meetings with other leaders, I soon realized we had a dilemma. Our relational initiatives were no longer practical. We were trying to keep our teams socially distanced to avoid the spread. In addition to that, mandates were coming out that we should not gather in large groups, soon changing from 100 to 50 and then to no more than 10 people. How could we be intentional and ensure that relationships and opportunities to support one another could continue? How could isolating our teams from one another help them thrive, much less survive? We had to revisit our plans.

While we created a website offering resources to support our team's mental health and post-COVID-19 education, it felt incomplete. So much was transitioning to a virtual platform, such as patient care, team meetings, and even the COVID-19 updates. Comfort levels with technology were growing, but how can you ensure that the connections we were having were beneficial and effective? We asked many questions, but in the long run, it would have to be a trial-and-error plan.

With a pretty robust team across our system who were used to rounding in the outpatient offices and offering spiritual support to physicians, APPs, and staff, they quickly transitioned to a virtual platform. They would connect through Microsoft Teams with individuals and groups to check in on their well-being. Some of them connected from the outpatient office, while others who were transitioned to working from home connected from there. At times, our team led a themed devotional or prayer for that clinical team prior to their daily huddle and workday— anything we could offer as support was greatly appreciated. We kept the time to a minimum so that it would not become a burden, but we wanted to offer them an opportunity to share their mission moments, experiences, and concerns and just check in on them. Physicians in some of our regions were more connected than in other regions, so supporting some of the less connected was difficult to guarantee. In other areas, our team had built strong relationships with the physicians, so connecting was easier. Every region had to figure out the best way to communicate with their clinical teams.

Our quarterly Finding Meaning in Medicine® connections came to a halt. Our teams sought the best ways to ensure our physicians connected and felt heard. With an opportunity to turn the typical in-person meeting into a virtual setting, many of our physician champions pushed back; they didn't want to do this virtually. Many wanted to wait and regroup when in-person meetings could happen safely again. However, some embraced this newfound opportunity to reach physician colleagues who may not have been able to participate previously. We had to bridge that gap somehow, and that meant readjusting the plans, again.

Being a part of a large system made it difficult to create a one-size-fits-all program. As much as we could, programs were developed with the opportunity for each of those regions to adjust them to fit the needs of their local team. Different opportunities were available in every location, and timing was based on whether that region was in a surge or planning for a surge. So, while some could arrange opportunities for the teams to connect, others couldn't spare the time.

Prior to a surge in the area of one of our hospitals, leadership invited a group of physicians to lunch in a socially distanced, large conference room and offered them the opportunity to share their concerns. Although this team had not experienced many COVID patients at the time, they did share the experiences their physician family members or friends had described. They spoke about their anxiety of waiting for the "flood of patients." Leadership was there to listen and support. I was told physicians from that group asked if they could meet again because it helped them process their fears and concerns.

Transitioning to Virtual Coaching at Avera Health

Until recently, I believed the best way to counsel and coach was face-to-face. As a licensed professional counselor, I had been trained to do the psychosocial assessment in person to ensure I was catching every verbal and nonverbal cue. I enjoyed this in-person luxury for five years before COVID-19 changed it all. I was then forced to do my first, and every, coaching session via Zoom. With time, I made this unfamiliar format into one that I actually enjoyed. It was effective. People felt better. It saved time and money. However, I did feel guilty that I wasn't seeing my clients in person when they were so dedicated to caring for their own patients face-to-face.

I created a calm and soothing home office environment. But I felt anything but calm during my first few Zoom sessions. My expectations were high that these interactions would be as warm and engaging through a screen. I had to console hurts and tears over video, which seemed cold, hopefully only to me.

I felt the challenge of the virtual format more than ever as I listened to a physician talk about having three patients die of COVID-19 in a day and then receiving a call that her grandmother had passed away. There was so much grief, loss, and disappointment to process virtually.

Processing critical incidents over Zoom was my biggest adjustment. How could I express my sadness, validate their emotions, and move them toward a stronger, more resilient place to take on the next incident? No hugs, no wiping tears, just doing the very best I could to give comfort and encourage grace, while instilling hope and courage.

It was easier to build connections on Zoom than I had thought. I did have to work a bit harder on connecting and being present. Initially, I also got distracted by worrying about how I looked on camera. An unexpected downside of Zoom was that it often interrupted my hoodie, yoga pants, ponytail, and no-makeup days.

Physician Stories of Virtual Coaching at Avera Health

COVID-19 pushed us to make Zoom comfortable. Many physicians even preferred this format.

One Avera physician shared:

> I don't consider myself an anxious person. And I am pretty used to working in controlled chaos. So, when COVID-19 hit our area, I was somewhat surprised at how I felt. I was looking at projections that were unbelievable, being told I may have to see these patients with inadequate PPE and maybe even a bandana, thinking I may have to make extremely difficult decisions about which of my patients would get resources such as ventilators and, in some cases, telling them I had nothing to offer and sending them home to die. At the same time, we were learning of many health care workers becoming very ill and even dying. I worried that my children would grow up without a parent or that I would bring this illness home to my family. I was quarantining myself away from my family, making me even more isolated from the people who bring me joy. My colleagues at work were stressed, and we didn't know if we were going to see enormous amounts of patients, while possibly losing income due to closing down of elective procedures and clinics.
>
> The unknown is often so difficult to deal with, as there is no direction to fight, and I felt I had little control over what was to happen. I reached out to Mary Wolf from the LIGHT program. We arranged a Zoom meeting to just talk about what was happening and how I felt. The Zoom format allowed us to meet frequently without masks and travel time. It helped me to have someone to talk to who works with physicians and providers and understands our unique work environment. I was given permission to feel anxious about what was happening and that so many were also having these similar feelings.

I had to separate what I could control and what I could not. We also talked a lot about self-care and trying to find ways to be healthy and find the silver lining in a lot of chaos. We met weekly for several weeks, and as we continued to prepare for a storm, I felt more prepared and stronger to face it. I feel like now I am more ready and confident that I have the tools to not only do my job but also to care for my family and ask for what I need.

Another Avera physician shared this:

I've been so pleased with my physician coaching sessions over Zoom. As a rural physician, I would not be able to participate without this kind of technology, given the distance required for in-person meetings. And I was pleasantly surprised with how easily a relationship was built without meeting in person. This is far superior to just a voice phone call.

I think it's also good for the coach, too. They can see me in my home, in my natural habitat, so to speak. The risks related to COVID-19 are mitigated for my family, and I can talk with my coach without wearing a mask. Most important, I've benefited tremendously from executive coaching. I'm able to enjoy a good work-life balance and be more productive with better quality of life. My wife and children have noticed the positive changes. To me, that might be the most meaningful measure.

Challenges / Best Practices for AdventHealth

While moving to a virtual setting had it challenges, we have learned and continue to learn a lot. Engagement has to be more intentional, strategic, and prioritized. It was easy to disappear from a meeting with just the click of a button. How do you involve everyone on the virtual call to offer their thoughts, opinions, and experiences? How do you ensure that one person is not overtaking the conversation because it's hard to read the virtual "room"? How do you manage the "you're on mute," "can you please mute yourself when you are not speaking," and "do you hear feedback on your end?" commentary that happens during **every, single meeting**? It takes practice, and it takes setting up expectations and reminders in the beginning, but it definitely requires a lot more effort than it did before. This is no longer about a call to share information and talk "at" people. They won't hear you. There are too many distractions taking them away from the conversation.

Another challenge we faced while redesigning programming and even developing resources to support our teams was the underutilization of those resources. It took creativity and continuous evaluation to ensure we were meeting their needs.

Whether it's a virtual counseling session or a meeting, you must stay engaged and not get distracted with a ding from your phone or a pop-up email on your computer. It is noticeable and will distract from the conversation and the opportunity to build that relationship.

Along with the challenges, we do grow, and we can find benefits to using the virtual setting. In many cases, we can reach more people. For our physicians who live farther away and don't want to extend their day another hour or so, jumping onto a virtual meeting from home helped them connect when they couldn't previously.

Large meetings and conferences also transitioned to a virtual platform. In some cases, there was a freeze on attending conferences, regardless of their online accessibility. However, more opportunities were available for physicians and leadership to participate in meetings and conferences since they could connect easily from their office or the comfort of their home. There were no travel costs and no travel time for which to account in their schedules. The virtual setting does offer a lot more convenience to already busy individuals.

Silver Linings of Virtual Care at Avera Health

While there are limitations of virtual care, I noticed myself focusing more on the blessings. I was grateful to still be able to coach my clients and be there during their tough days.

- ⊙ Zoom also allowed me to know my colleagues and clients better, including chatting with their children and meeting their pets.
- ⊙ I learned technology, and so did my clients. I'm glad that virtual care pushed me to be a more adaptable counselor and coach. My clients and I have post-trauma growth for sure.
- ⊙ It forced me to find meaning in the madness. Who did I want to become? What changes did I want to make?
- ⊙ I worked from home. Even though I worked longer hours during the COVID-19 months, I loved having my 16-year-old son and my husband just a room away.

Well-being didn't stop. Just like everything else, we did a workaround. Luckily, love and kindness transmit over Zoom.

Conclusion

The virtual setting was not new, and it is definitely not going away anytime soon. Through this transition to a virtual platform, we learned grace for ourselves and others as we created a new well-being strategy by trial and error. Through this, we also learned that it isn't essential to have the right answer the first time. We need to adjust, review our plans, and, if necessary, redesign what we have to best support our teams.

DeAnna Santana-Cebollero, PhD
Director, Physician Well-Being and Engagement
AdventHealth

Mary Wolf, MS, LPC-MH
Director, LIGHT Program
Avera Medical Group

Endnotes

1. Wysockey-Johnson D. Collegiality and Physician Well-Being. In: Dianne E. McCallister TH, ed. *Transforming the Heart of Practice: An Organizational and Personal Approach to Physician Well-being*: Springer 2019:155.

CHAPTER 9

HEALTH CARE DELIVERY IN A POST-COVID-19 WORLD

Robert Rodgers, MD

Introduction

When the ball dropped in Times Square as the clock struck midnight on January 1, 2020, those of us in health care had no idea what was in store for us over the ensuing months. Everything seemed normal as we tried to recall the words of "Auld Lang Syne" and sing along with our family and friends to welcome in the new year. Few knew that a report to the World Health Organization (WHO) had been filed earlier that New Year's Eve which reported a cluster of pneumonia cases in Wuhan, China, that had occurred with no known etiology.[1] We headed to work the next day focused on the patients who entrusted us to partner with them in their health journey and continued on our controlled cadence of innovation that we hoped would lead us to processes and technologies that would allow us to improve our whole-person care delivery.

Our environment changed quickly, though, and by January 7, the WHO had identified a new virus that it called COVID-19.[2] By month's end, cases were reported in multiple countries, including the United States, and the number of fatalities was rising at an alarming rate. March brought an expanded spread of the virus that extended to the point that a pandemic was declared, and international travel bans were implemented. Hospital systems in places like New York City were quickly overextended and scrambling to find needed ventilators and personal protective equipment (PPE). Almost overnight, nothing in health care was "normal." Patients were suddenly afraid to leave their homes to seek routine care, tents popped up outside of hospital emergency departments in anticipation of large volumes of those sick with the virus, and health care organizations focused on finding additional personnel and the PPE needed to keep them safe. Current strategies were pushed aside while rapid decision groups and command centers became the norm. This pandemic quickly shifted priorities and allowed for transformations that would accelerate changes in health care for the care delivery teams, large health care systems, and patients. In many ways, this terrible pandemic has been the catalyst needed to initiate changes in our system that are now benefiting both patients and those delivering the care. In this chapter, we will highlight some of those prominent changes and how the health care system was able to flex the ability to adapt during the pandemic and accelerate needed change that would not have occurred in this expedited time frame had the "normal" we were accustomed to remained.

The Ability to Change

Albert Einstein is quoted as saying, "The measure of intelligence is the ability to change." Those I observed leading the way in health care delivery certainly displayed a high level of this intelligence as they quickly reacted to the needs of patients and providers in response to this pandemic. Routine scheduled meetings were cleared, which allowed teams to review and act on information received from emergency departments, hospitals, physician offices, and patients. Out of these structured work groups sprang the initiatives that have changed how care is delivered and received at a pace not seen previously. Let's first examine how things changed in our acute care facilities—the emergency rooms and hospitals.

Stories and pictures of patients suffering from COVID-19 infections and those caring for them preceded the official announcement of the pandemic in March of 2020. Local hospitals worried that their personnel, PPE, and other resources would not be adequate to meet the anticipated surge of infected patients. Compounding this uncertainty was the deficiency in reliable data on transmission of the virus and recommended treatments because the recommendations from the Center for Disease Control (CDC) seemed to change daily. With this ever-changing background in place, change began. First, emergency rooms changed how they handled all patients. Screening measures, including temperature checks and risk-stratifying questionnaires, were implemented outside the doors of the emergency room. Specifically, dedicated areas of care for those at risk and those known to be COVID-19 positive were established. This was done to improve care for patients with the virus and to prevent exposure to those seeking treatment in the emergency department for other reasons. Despite quickly implementing this type of triage, a generalized fear of going to the emergency room, even for potentially serious conditions, arose in the community. In June, the Advisory Board reported numbers at 70 percent of consumers who were very or somewhat concerned about contracting the virus if they were to go to emergency room facilities to receive care. This translated into lower rates of hospitalizations for acute conditions like heart attacks, strokes, and appendicitis. In a release on June 12, the CDC reported that in April 2020, there was a 42 percent decrease in emergency room visits overall.[3] Hospital systems like AdventHealth continued to work with their emergency department teams to ensure they were safe places to visit for those who truly needed emergency care. Even with these specific interventions, volumes only increased slowly and continued to be below the pre-COVID-19 numbers through the third quarter of 2020. With the number of COVID-19 patients requiring hospitalization increasing, other options for care needed to be considered. The expansion of home monitoring became an integral part of the emergency room acute care setting because it allowed for sick yet stable patients to receive care in the comfort of their own home, while allowing hospital beds to be reserved for those with more severe symptoms.

Inside the hospital itself, life was also different. As the number of COVID-19 cases increased, systems expanded intensive care unit (ICU) capacity and searched for more ventilators so patients suffering from pneumonia and respiratory failure could be treated appropriately. Clinical teams led by physicians consistently updated care pathways based on the latest available data. Those performing the direct care of the patients were at a high risk of becoming infected themselves and initially faced a shortage of appropriate PPE because in-stock supplies quickly ran low.

Despite this increased risk, care team members continued to deliver the compassionate care each patient deserves. These frontline caregivers were true heroes. Most hospitals pivoted to segregating COVID-19 patients in designated wards and ICUs as need dictated. This set the stage for better care by having specialized teams specifically trained to care for these patients. Visitation policies were changed, and soon no visitors were allowed in the hospitals. This created a new problem, that of isolation. Patients felt alone without the support of their friends and family, while family members felt helpless and out of touch with what was happening to their loved ones inside the hospital walls. System changes quickly followed to leverage video technology, which allowed connection to continue between the family and the patient. Often, daily video visits with family members were scheduled, which kept the lines of communication open and facilitated the formation of a bond with the care team. The family looked forward to these calls each day as they waited for an update on their loved one. The calls were done when the patient could be a part of the call or even when they were unconscious and on a ventilator.

Despite the utilization of video technology in this fashion, too many patients died without family members by their side. The need to dedicate staff to caring for COVID-19 patients and the need to ration PPE resources required a shift in other services offered in the hospital. Many states put mandates in place to postpone elective surgeries in order to save precious PPE, decrease the rate of spread of the virus, and improve surgical outcomes. Studies like the one published in *The Lancet* showed a significant increase in mortality for routine surgeries when the patient was found to be COVID-19 positive.[4] Although patients understood the reasoning behind the delay in their elective procedure, accepting another 8–12 week delay for a nonurgent orthopedic or other elective surgery was often difficult.

Hospital/ER Post-COVID-19 Health Care Changes

1. Daily screenings for elevated temperatures done on all visitors and staff
2. Specifically designated areas for care of COVID-19 patients in the emergency room, hospital, and ICU

3. Limitation set on the number of visitors allowed per patient admitted to the hospital and leveraging video technology for family visits when needed

4. All hospital employees had to wear surgical masks, and those in areas of direct patient contact added face shields and other appropriate PPE

5. Increased utilization of telemedicine/video visits to address emergency room needs

6. Incorporation of increased in-home monitoring and hospital at-home services

7. Increased dedication of resources to the supply chain team to assure no shortage of needed PPE, testing kits, and other supplies

Outside of the acute care setting in physician offices and urgent care centers, changes were also occurring at a dizzying pace. First, rapid changes were made to assure the physician office was a safe place for both the patients and the care team. This included new sterilization techniques after each patient and dedicated exam rooms for evaluating sick patients. Waiting rooms were suddenly large, vacant spaces, as the individual car was where the waiting took place until it was time for the doctor to see the patient. Electronic check-in processes were designed to allow patients to schedule appointments, register, scan insurance cards, and pay online without ever entering the office. Then, when it was time for their appointment, a simple text alerted them that their room was ready and to please come inside.

Urgent care and primary care offices also found patients could be tested for the virus without coming into the office and exposing other patients or staff. Drive-up testing centers became the norm and were extremely popular with patients.

The most dramatic change seen in the ambulatory space was how the pandemic catalyzed the rapid adoption of telehealth. Many systems had initiated utilizing this technology prior to COVID-19, but only in small volumes and most commonly around an urgent care application. With states implementing stay-at-home orders, this innovative form of care, including both telephonic and video visits, became a necessity. The previous barrier of reimbursement was pushed aside as clinicians did what they had to do to care for their patients. Fortunately, the Centers for Medicare and Medicaid Services (CMS) (followed by most commercial insurance companies) quickly made exceptions to the established rules that allowed for adjustments in reimbursement, making the telehealth visit financially comparable to face-to-face visits of the same complexity. In an article entitled, "Telehealth transformation: COVID-19 and the rise of virtual care," the authors from Duke University School of Medicine reported that in a four-week period, the share of telehealth visits at their institution increased from less than 1 percent to 70 percent of total visits.[5] This was not unique to Duke, as comparable numbers were reported around the country. This advancement seems to be here to stay because the medical community has found that many conditions can be treated with the same quality through a video visit as they can in the office. Certainly, some patient concerns cannot be addressed telephonically due to their seriousness or complexity, and there are times when there is no substitution for a detailed and focused physical exam, but the benefits these video visits provide are undeniable. The televisit could evolve into the modern-day house call, as telemedicine is simply an alternative care delivery model. The same quality standards and outcomes will be expected as the patient or provider selects this option.

This advancement in the telehealth care delivery model will benefit both care providers and patients. The results will include increased physician access, increased convenience for patients, and significant time savings. However, this is only part of the outpatient changes that are taking place. "The Doctor Won't See You Now," was the headline of an article in the *Wall Street Journal* on September 11, 2020. In this article, Laura Landro described how primary care was moving toward teams of health care professionals that may not always include a physician or face-to-face interaction. In the article she states, "The COVID-19 pandemic is accelerating this restructuring of primary care, which has been gathering steam for years."[6] In the team approach, telephonic, video, and in-person contacts with the patients will occur more frequently and with a variety of specialized team members. The physician will still be directing the care based on the patient's personal health goals, but a variety of resources in and outside the office will be connected to deliver exactly what each patient needs. The connection made in the typical face-to-face visit between the patient and the physician will continue to be a driving factor in maintaining a certain level of the in-person visits because they are important to facilitate a sense of trust between the two parties.

Ambulatory Post-COVID-19 Health Care Changes

1. Removal of the traditional waiting room filled with patients
2. Increased leverage on telemedicine/video visits for assessing acute needs, chronic disease management, and preventive medicine
3. Increasing online services to include appointments, registration, and payment

4. Daily temperature screening for all employees and patients accessing the office
5. Clinic staff all wearing surgical masks, and providers also adding face shields
6. Multiple patient options to consult with provider, therefore increasing access and convenience
7. More physicians now allotting some of their time to working from home

The financial impact the pandemic has had on the health care industry has been widely publicized. The COVID-19 effect on the economics of health care was also profound. An article in *JAMA* reported that 62 percent of physicians surveyed had their salaries reduced, and some offices reported a decrease in patient volumes by as much as 75 percent.[7] At a higher level, the American Hospital Association has reported that hospitals and health care systems around the country were projected to lose more than $200 billion between March 1 and June 30 due to the pandemic.[8] Our own AdventHealth was not immune to this and reported losses close to $263 million over this time period. With most physician practices and health systems depending on volume of services for the majority of their incoming revenue stream, predetermined budgets for 2020 were necessarily discarded. The apprehension patients felt, which kept them quarantined at home, drastically decreased the volumes of not only our emergency rooms, but also physician offices. Many physicians in private practice settings grounded mostly in a fee-for-service world were suddenly struggling to meet payroll and keep the doors open. CMS advanced payments and payroll protection loans helped many for a short period as they waited for volumes to increase. At the same time, those providers and organizations that had already ventured into the risk world reaped the benefits of the decreased utilization that was occurring and watched as their profit margins grew. This dichotomy caused many to step back and reanalyze their individual market strategies, leading to an intentional decision to speed up plans to increase their exposure in the risk world. Thus, the pandemic became the impetus for deployment of a diversification strategy that would include more full risk.

Conclusion

It is obvious, as we now reflect on the COVID-19 pandemic, how necessary alterations in traditional health care delivery occurred rapidly to meet the needs of both patients and care delivery teams. Most of these changes have improved the patient experience and will continue to be a part of our systems moving forward. More rigorous screening procedures, video visits, online registrations, and movement of expanded medical services to the home will help to decrease cost while increasing convenience and quality of care moving forward. Throughout this period, one concept that resurfaced was that of trust. We all have a fear of the unknown and of things we do not control, and this is exactly what most consumers face when accessing health care, especially when a pandemic is raging. By developing and implementing inventive workflows and processes, health care systems and care delivery teams have been able to recapture the trust of the general public and thus decrease this anxiety and allow for routine chronic disease management, preventive care, and emergency care to resume. "There are far better things ahead than any we leave behind," C.S. Lewis stated. The pandemic showed us the importance of remembering this and reminded us all how we must constantly be willing to reevaluate our long-established traditions in health care and be open to new thinking and new alternatives that will launch us to the next level of patient care. The arrival of the COVID-19 virus was able to press the launch button for us in 2020, but now we need to continue this trajectory of open-mindedness because it is what our care teams and patients deserve.

Robert Rodgers, MD
Vice President, Senior Care
AdventHealth

Endnotes

1. Joost WW, Andrew R, C. CA, J. PS, C. PH. Pathophysiology, Transmission, Diagnosis, and Treatment of Coronavirus Disease 2019 (COVID-19): A Review. *JAMA*. 2020;324(8):782-793.

2. Organization WH. Archived: WHO Timeline-COVID-19. https://www.wsj.com/articles/the-new-doctors-appointment-11599662314. Published 2020. Accessed.

3. Hartnett K, Kite-Powell A, DeVies J, et al. Impact of the COVID-19 Pandemic on Emergency Department Visits - United States, January 1, 2019-May 30, 2020. *MMWR Morbidity and Mortality Weekly Report*. 2020;69(23):699-704.

4. Nepogodiev D, Bhangu A, Glasbey JC, et al. Mortality and pulmonary complications in patients undergoing surgery with perioperative SARS-CoV-2 infection: an international cohort study. *The Lancet*. 2020;396(10243):27-38.

5. Jedrek W, Marat F, Blake C, et al. Telehealth transformation: COVID-19 and the rise of virtual care. *Journal of the American Medical Informatics Association*. 2020;27(6):957-962.

6. Landro L. The Doctor Won't See You Now. *Wall Street Journal*2020.

7. Rubin R. COVID-19's Crushing Effects on Medical Practices, Some of Which Might Not Survive. *JAMA*. 2020;324(4):321-323.

8. Association AH. Hospitals and Health Systems Face Unprecedented Financial Pressures Due to COVID-19. https://www.aha.org/system/files/media/file/2020/05/aha-covid19-financial-impact-0520-FINAL.pdf. Published 2020. Accessed.

PART II

BUILDING RESILIENCE

ORGANIZATIONAL CULTURE MATTERS

Good doctors are bad patients: good at caring for others, bad about caring for themselves. Doctors tend to ignore or deny their symptoms, self-diagnose and self-treat, invite "sidewalk consults," and only seek true professional help when other options are exhausted. It is becoming progressively clear that organizational commitment and involvement are highly beneficial, if not essential, in addressing physician burnout and reducing unanticipated turnover. Engaged senior administrators take an active role in addressing the health and well-being of the core medical staff of the institution—understanding the issues, investing resources in strategies to effect open communication, building trust, and moving assertively to resolve apparent problems.

CHAPTER 10

SHIFTING THE CULTURE OF PHYSICIAN VULNERABILITIES: CONVERSATIONS ON MORAL INJURY AND RACISM

Tyon L. Hall, PhD
Tania Aylmer, LMHC

For what may seem like obvious reasons, the psychological wellness of physicians is essential. Many areas of a health care organization are impacted when the physician is struggling. A distraught physician can affect team morale, increase medical errors, and place an organization at risk for litigation issues. More importantly, a struggling physician can be at risk of harm to themselves.

While most issues are kept private, there are times when a community or, in this case, a nation collectively experiences trauma. During those times, health care organizations must become flexible and open to shifting conversations to ensure that physicians have what they need to do the necessary work. We joined the AdventHealth team in the spring of 2020. As new employees, we immersed ourselves with onboarding, completing the required training, and getting our offices and schedules just right. These tasks may seem familiar for new hires and usually are familiar; however, shifts were occurring in our health care and social climate that would abruptly put a stop to what we knew as typical. With over 30 years of collective mental health experience, nothing could have prepared us to manage the personal responses and challenges of 2020 while offering emotional support to those on the front lines in health care.

On May 25, 2020, George Floyd, a 46-year-old African American male, was killed in Minneapolis, Minnesota, by police officers for allegedly using a counterfeit bill. This killing ignited worldwide protests combating police brutality and systemic racism. By the end of June 2020, the coronavirus had taken the lives of 126,140 people in the United States, and there were 2.59 million confirmed cases in the States. These crisis events affected our health care system culture emotionally, physically, and socially. In this chapter, we hope to share our experience of tough conversations during health care and social crises.

We were redeployed in July 2020 to provide emotional support to the COVID-19 units. Between the two of us, we covered four campuses. Our goal was to check in with as many clinical and nonclinical staff as possible to offer self-care strategies, connect staff to resources, and ultimately let staff know that the administration cares. We heard similar challenges that other health care systems have written about, including shortages of personal protective equipment (PPE), staff turnover, and overall emotional exhaustion. By conducting these mental health rounds, we were reminded of the value of leaning into tough conversations and the importance of vulnerability.

Conversations on Moral Injury

Research outlines that prolonged emotional exhaustion can often result in burnout, compassion fatigue, anxiety, depression, post-traumatic stress disorder, and moral injury.[1] In times of crisis and this most recent pandemic, vulnerabilities are exposed and can reveal opportunities for change as an individual and as an organization. Individually, a crisis reveals psychological difficulties. Crises show us which procedures, processes, and functions are working smoothly and which ones need attention. Many organizations faced challenging problems, such as supporting the medical and ancillary staff's mental health as they responded to the public health crisis.

Moral injury is a deep sense of transgression, including feelings of shame, grief, meaninglessness, and remorse, from having violated core moral beliefs and is also a betrayal of what's right by someone who holds legitimate authority in a high-stakes situation.[2] We saw firsthand the trauma our providers were living day in and day out as well as the grief. Clinical staff worked extended hours, spent time researching the latest information about COVID-19 on their off-hours, and worried about protecting themselves and their families from the virus. A high volume of patients and high acuity of care meant long and exhausting days.

Staffing posed a challenge in which nurses and physicians were pulled from various units to accommodate the high demands. These medical personnel also experienced moral distress around patient deaths, resource allocation, and a fear of scarcity. Additionally, we heard talks on economic insecurity, social and family life disruption, stigmatization of being a health care worker, and overall a sense of powerlessness. For many, their only contact with their home support systems was through video chats and phone calls; ultimately, the power of touch and connection decreased.

Some research surrounding physician burnout suggests a health professional is at fault for their emotional state; they aren't resilient enough and need to learn to recover better. Yet moral injury means something larger is at play. Because we experience moral injury when we face an incongruency between personal values and policies, we must consider a systemic perspective to shifting change. If this mindset can change, the results would be immense, and health care professionals could thrive.[3]

Discussing moral injury allows clinicians to express what the burnout label failed to describe—the agony of being frequently locked in double binds when every choice one makes yields a compromised outcome and when each decision contradicts the reason for years of sacrifice. As a result, many experienced the well-understood symptoms of burnout, and they kept burning out, in defiance of the many and well-meaning interventions designed to combat it. The burnout epidemic continues unabated because the moral injury at the root of the problem remains unaddressed. Burnout is the symptom, but moral injury may be the cause.[3]

Change needs to happen in all health care system arenas, including clinicians, health care administrators, policymakers, patients, and families. However, a great starting point is having hard conversations addressing burnout and moral injury. One approach to accomplish this is to accept vulnerability as a cultural norm—ideally, creating a vulnerability culture where one can admit they have a need, then feel safe to reach out for support. Health care workers traditionally have been reluctant to ask for help because vulnerability is deeply attached to shame and not courage. Physicians would rather bear the burden alone than admit to hardship because they believe it is weak.

Brené Brown, professor, author, and researcher studying courage, vulnerability, shame, and empathy, defines vulnerability as the courage to be imperfect and the compassion to be kind to yourself and then to others. Vulnerability is the birthplace of love, belonging, joy, courage, empathy, and creativity.[4] We deflect feeling vulnerable by striving for perfection, numbing out, disrupting joyful moments by imagining all the ways things could go wrong. We do whatever we can to avoid feelings of shame, anxiety, uncertainty, and fear. Vulnerability is hard, it feels uncomfortable, but it pushes us toward a place of authenticity and our truth.

How do we begin stepping into a space of vulnerability? Start with being mindful. Adopting a practice of openness and awareness of your environment and your own thoughts, feelings, and triggers will help you recognize when you're disengaged because you're afraid. Next, don't stuff your emotions. Become self-aware. Recognize that facing vulnerability takes a huge amount of courage. Show up, face the fear, and move forward. Seek excellence, not perfection. Strive to be yourself and connect with what you were specifically created to do. There are many benefits to being vulnerable. It helps build connections in relationships, leads to authenticity in the physician-patient relationship, increases self-worth, aids innovation and motivation, provokes compassion, is a call for accountability, and means less loneliness.

Conversations on Race

While health care staff were challenged with managing their professional emotions due to COVID-19, they also had to contend with personal feelings related to racial tensions in the community and tough conversations in the workplace. On June 2, 2020, our CEO sent out a message to all employees entitled, "Silence Is Not an Option." In the statement, he noted, "There is unimaginable hurt in our black communities given the long history of such senseless deaths, including the recent killings of Mr. Floyd in Minnesota, Ahmaud Arbery in Georgia, and Breonna Taylor in Kentucky. We cannot remain bystanders. While there is breath in us, silence is not an option . . . To deliver compassionate,

Christ-like care, we must preserve and advocate for the safety of others. We must love beyond borders, skin colors, and cultural barriers. We must own it and think carefully about what role we can play in bringing about change."

For many, this served as an opportunity to begin and continue conversations that are vulnerable and uncomfortable. Addressing racial emotions in the workplace is difficult but necessary to create a psychologically safe workplace. Research on racial emotions proposes that many workers expect to experience negative emotions from an interracial interaction.[5] The interaction's anxiety can lead to unhealthy strategies such as hostility, antagonism, and avoidance.[6] However, these responses can change based on the individuals' perceived openness, and an alternative strategy can be implemented.

The Center for Physician Wellbeing had the privilege of witnessing meaningful interracial interactions. We facilitated a mini discussion that integrated issues of the COVID-19 pandemic and social unrest. We collaborated with Mission and Ministry and titled the presentation, "Building Bridges During Times of Crisis." The presentation covered several areas that addressed elements of conducting a healthy conversation.

Rather than avoidance, research shows that when individuals choose to engage in conversation, it can lead to more positive impressions of interracial interactions.[6] There are several stages of having conversations on race. These stages include preparation, encounter, engagement, and execution.[7]

Dr. Hardy believes that engagement occurs after preparation and encounter. Preparation refers to didactics or teachings, while encounter entails creating a "safe space" environmentally and emotionally in which to engage.[7] Once these areas have been developed and implemented, execution can take place in a deeper and more meaningful way for all involved.

In the health care arena, preparation could include mandatory trainings on race, discrimination, and unconscious bias. Many peers have discussed taking the Harvard Project Implicit Test. This test allows you to see categories in which you may have biases, including gender, race, and skin tone. AdventHealth has implemented several educational opportunities, formally and informally, through the learning network and team sharing.

As an organization, the encounter stage is equally as important as the preparation stage. Creating a safe space refers to both psychological and environmental safety. Organizations must ensure that areas represent diversity and should call attention to the importance of the conversation as our CEO did in his letter. These changes may include updating pictures and art that reflect the community the organization serves as well as frequent reminders to value differences and encourage empathy.

Once training is complete and the invitation and space is prepped, engaging in an open and honest discussion can proceed. Real engagement on race and racism requires vulnerability and being okay to be uncomfortable. Execution is critical to make connections. Thus, having compassion for one another's experience and providing a sense of visibility and importance creates a road toward trust.

To shift the culture toward authenticity, we have to be vulnerable and courageous. We have the power to make a difference, one difficult conversation about moral injury or race at a time. Be the one to create a safe place for colleagues to feel comfortable sharing their hardships personally and professionally. Create the atmosphere where it is okay to not be okay, then take action to be a part of the solution.

Tyon L. Hall, PhD
Manager/Psychotherapist
The Center for Physician Well-Being
AdventHealth Orlando

Tania Aylmer, LMHC
Manager, Clinical Professionalism
AdventHealth Orlando

Endnotes

1. Su J, Shen L, Chen H. Maintaining Mental Health among Medical Staff during the COVID-19 Pandemic: Taiwan's Experience. *Journal of the Formosan Medical Association = Taiwan yi zhi.* 2020.

2. Koenig HG, Youssef NA, Pearce M. Assessment of Moral Injury in Veterans and Active Duty Military Personnel With PTSD: A Review. *Frontiers in Psychiatry.* 2019;10.

3. Talbot SG, Dean W. Physicians Aren't 'Burning Out.' They're Suffering from Moral Injury. *Stat.* 2018;7(26):18.

4. Brené Brown. https://brenebrown.com/ Accessed.

5. Green TK. Racial Emotion in the Workplace. *Southern California Law Review.* 2013;86, 959.

6. Trawalter S, Richeson J, Shelton J. Predicting Behavior during Interracial Interactions: A Stress and Coping Approach. *Personality and Social Psychology Review: An Official Journal of the Society for Personality and Social Psychology, Inc.* 2009;13(4):243-268.

7. Hardy K. Race Inside and Outside the Therapy Room. In. Washington, D.C.: Psychotherapy Networker Symposium; 2015.

CHAPTER 11

THE DOCTOR AND THE SYSTEM: THE NEED FOR TRUST AND COLLABORATION

Dianne McCallister, MD, MBA

Introduction

The impact of the COVID-19 pandemic of 2020 has been vast across economic, personal, scientific, and political arenas. One developing issue is the spiritual crisis impacting physician well-being. The calling of physicians to help others and to use science is the root of physician spirituality. Even prior to the pandemic, this was often done at personal expense. The spirituality of physicians has been pushed to the limit during the pandemic by multiple factors including the rapid spread of the virus, the surge volumes of patients, failures in previous pandemic preparation, missteps in communication at local and national levels, and overwhelmed administrative leadership in some organizations. A crisis of physical, emotional, and spiritual well-being has emerged. The physical and emotional demands will ease and will leave well-documented post-traumatic stress disorder (PTSD) of a spiritual nature that has been well documented in other, smaller crises. Well-being science has described easily implemented measures that create a safety net. Physicians and other clinicians need ongoing spiritual and emotional support in anticipation of a "spiritual crisis" as they recover from the physical impacts of the pandemic.

The Global Pandemic of 2020 has affected the health care world in many dimensions. Supply chain limitations and vulnerabilities, staffing shortages, rapid-cycle research, and vaccine development and political unrest have all shaken the foundations that support operations at the time when care is most needed. While the focus of administrators and individual health care providers has been necessarily focused on these basics of day-to-day operations, a crisis has been developing.

Interviews with over 2,000 physicians internationally over a decade[1] and similar conversations with nurses, EMTs, and other clinical professions revealed two primary reasons they chose a health care career: (1) a desire to help people, and (2) a love of science. People often choose a career, particularly in the service sector, for "meaning and purpose," perhaps better described as the "spirituality of work." As the COVID-19 pandemic unfolded, the seeds of a spiritual crisis were sown. The inability to help patients has been a source of great moral distress. The science was not yet in place to meet the needs of the patients, and the overwhelmed system capacity prevented the ability to deliver best-known practice of care. With neither adequate resources nor established science to lean upon, health care workers experienced distress. Compounding this, a disconnect between urgency at the front line and the limited ability of health care administration to respond created a chasm of distrust. This crisis of trust appears to be more pronounced in facilities without meaningful and efficient two-way communication and in which administrative leadership fails to listen to the urgent needs of frontline workers, or worse, threatens staff for expressing real and urgent concern.

If quality of care, business efficiencies, need for a supportive culture, and ongoing intellectual growth are viewed as the "machinery" of well-being, then spiritual/emotional support can be viewed as the "oil" that keeps the machine from seizing. Without the "oil" of emotional/spiritual support, the clinical "machinery" creates friction, overheats, and grinds to a halt.

Personal Factors

Since the two primary reasons physicians go into medicine are to help others and because they like science,[1] in spiritual language, this is the "calling" of the physician. Over half of participating physicians affirmed that they knew, before the age of 18, that medicine was their calling. As one physician put it, "I was born to be a physician. I don't remember a time when I did not know that." This reflects a vocation held close to the heart. In difficult times, staying connected to one's calling, the "why" of the profession, helps one cope. It helps physicians endure rigorous 12- to 14-hour days, face life-and-death situations, resolve difficult interactions with patients and families, and survive separation from their home life.[1]

During the pandemic, physicians have felt abandoned on many levels. In some cases, administrative support, for valid infection-prevention reasons, was removed from hospitals, thereby limiting communication and compromising the ability of administrators to personally view issues at the bedside. Shortages of personal protective equipment (PPE) created hazardous working conditions for physicians and staff who could not protect themselves from the disease they were fighting. And the virus was novel—meaning no established science protocol was available to guide treatment plans. Compounding these professional issues, many physicians moved out of their homes to prevent transmission of the virus to their families. As patient volume increased and physicians became ill or died, others took on additional workload to assure continuity of patient care, driving themselves to emotional and physical exhaustion.

In an attempt to control the uncontrollable, some administrators discouraged physicians from discussing their concerns, such as lack of PPE and other equipment and process issues, despite the reality that these issues were of deep concern.[2-4] This resulted in moral and psychological harm to already overtaxed physicians. Trust is betrayed when someone is put in a life-threatening situation with inadequate support and then their valid concerns dismissed. Declining transparency and denial of truth resulted in a breakdown of trust.

Volumes at peak surges of COVID-19 cases taxed system capabilities to the breaking point. For example, in New York City, 911 calls for cardiac arrest went from an average of 30 per day to 300 per day. This left physicians and other health care providers with very difficult decisions in regard to allocating resources, triaging care, and managing the burden of sickness and death.[5] The emotional impact of facing these decisions with or without adequate emotional support is significant.

One way to frame this crisis is through the lens of physician development and values instilled through training. Physicians are truth-seekers, problem-solvers. They are also competitive in the way they live out their calling to heal. Physicians take the Hippocratic Oath, which binds them to put aside their personal needs to care for the ill and wounded. In this pandemic, as in battlefield medicine, physicians are called on to assume personal danger to fulfill this oath.

Truth-Seekers. Physicians are trained to search for truth, seeking primary source information, and are trained to spot inconsistencies in data and logic, holding high the value of integrity.[6]

Problem Solvers. There were few clear answers or proven remedies for the new virus, yet patients were dying in large numbers. Resources available to treat patients safely (PPE, medications, etc.) were at a premium and were not under physician control. Some physicians obtained their own N95 PPE, which they were censured for using.[6]

Competitive. Physicians were competing with disease and death and concerned that their patient outcomes would be compared to those in other institutions with more resources and personnel.[6]

Hippocratic Oath. The tension between the oath to do no harm, the need for rapid innovation with unclear outcomes, and inadequate means to measure results of treatment weighed heavily on physicians in both academic and community settings.[7]

Personal Risk. Danger arises in many forms—personal danger of disease and death, inadequate PPE,[8-10] risk of infection, increased viral loads, exhaustion and fatigue from protracted disease surges, emotional danger from public shunning or from being isolated, professional danger—utilizing poorly understood treatment regimens due to lack of scientific evidence, public misinformation creating distrust of physicians/science, and high-visibility physician suicides from despair, fatigue, and hopelessness.[11-13]

Drivers of the Administrative/Clinical Chasm

1. Organizations may be faced with clinical demands exceeding their capacity and resources, including inadequate or expired supplies and equipment and untested processes.
2. Unreliable communication plans—although incident command structures are well-defined, organizations have been inconsistent in their attention to adequate drills to

assure that people in the organization are able to quickly fill roles and utilize processes as intended.

3. Organizational courage—the ability of the organization to listen carefully and respond to missteps and failures inherent in any complex situation.

4. Leadership styles—command and control over areas characterized by inadequate expertise and fear-based muzzling of communication versus courageous listening and honesty.

Societal Factors

During this pandemic and consistent with the Spanish flu pandemic of 1918,[14] significant societal issues have impacted the ability of the general public to assist in solving their own problems. This comes at the expense of frontline health care workers committed by their professional values to take care of all patients but who are overtaxed yet unable to care for themselves while performing their duties when clinical demands exceed the capacity of the system.

In speaking to physicians internationally and observing posts in social media, clearly the pandemic has been a wound in the very fabric of physicians' sense of meaning and purpose. We need to prevent further breakdown and hemorrhage by stitching up the wound.

Creating Solutions for a Spiritual Crisis

The spiritual nature of distress—physical, mental, social— must be dealt with as a critical factor in healing for physicians and caregivers, health care organizations, and society at large. Physician experience following the Aurora theater shootings of 2012 reveals a predictable pattern of PTSD approaching the anniversary of the event. Proactive conversations were facilitated to help physicians identify and acknowledge the source of anger and tension they were experiencing subconsciously. The COVID-19 pandemic is a crisis of international proportion, and the need to help physicians get in tune with their own feelings of anger, confusion, and despair should be initiated now to prevent a post-pandemic wave of despair.

Given the staggering pre-pandemic rate of physician suicide of 400 per year in the United States coupled with the highly publicized suicides of physicians during the pandemic sounds an alarm regarding the spiritual health of physicians. Properly implemented, systemic changes for physician well-being may create a pathway to further improvements that will benefit physicians in an ongoing manner. The four elements comprising the Medicus Integra© Award—Business and Quality, Cultural, Learning, and Resilience—may provide helpful guidance for ongoing physician support.

Personal Well-Being

On an individual level, the ability to acknowledge trauma, have a voice in decision-making, and receive explicit permission and a safe space to express anger and regret addresses a critical need in the healing of what can only be described as PTSD. Continued scientific advancement and training in the COVID-19 virus will provide a valid scientific base to support decision-making. In addition, public acknowledgement of the sacrifices made by clinicians, including efforts by patients and nonclinicians to express gratitude, are small but powerful antidotes to emotional and spiritual distress, helping physicians put their own sacrifice in the context of their calling. Finally, physicians need an opportunity to rest, to recover physically and emotionally.

Organizational/Administrative

Crisis communication and change management leaders have taught us the importance of acknowledging the challenges of the crisis, including responses that fail to adequately address the urgency or resources required. The framework for how such issues will be addressed in the future will create a bridge of trust. The inclusion of the physician voice in clinical decision-making and formal apologies when appropriate will only be feasible if there is emotional support and advanced leadership training to resolve misunderstandings and alleviate stress. A safe environment and respectful, honest communication will help rebuild trust.

- ⊙ **Communication.** Opportunities for clear communication have been abundant throughout the pandemic. Unfortunate issues common to crises, including evolving information and speculative misinformation, are compounded by evolving evidence. The ability of organizations to listen carefully to experts on the front line who were taking care of patients was sometimes hampered by enforced isolation of decision makers. Conversely, in organizations that were mindful of communication processes and tone, team members would state that this pandemic was "a huge growth in trust and skills" for the members of their team.
- ⊙ **Creating coalitions versus inciting fear/mistrust.** It is well known that the creation of coalitions and excellent change management diminish resistance to change. Organizations that used change management and incident control to create coalitions were able to quickly make needed changes. Organizations in

which leadership failed to use these well-described management techniques were more likely to create a culture of mistrust.

⊙ **Societal anger at restrictions.** As in the Spanish flu pandemic,[15] the balance between individual freedom and the common good was strained. In addition, the speed of onset resulted in major economic impact on individuals, families, and organizations and triggered raw emotions. The organization and provision of physical and emotional support was more often a hastily improvised system than a predetermined and tested system or process.

⊙ **Social media.** A new variable in this pandemic, social media allowed the rapid dissemination of critical information as well as the viral spread of intentional (or unintentional) misinformation. Adequate controls were not in place to alert the public to misinformation.

⊙ **Helping others.** Efforts to help others creates goodwill, while fear drives irrational behaviors. The hoarding of toilet paper is a benchmark illustration of irrational fear during the Pandemic of 2020.

Societal

Ongoing acknowledgment of the personal danger and sacrifice of frontline providers is a well-documented gift to honor the sacrifices of the few for the many. Examples range from verbal acknowledgement and certificates of appreciation to medals of honor and formal monuments honoring the professions.

Clearly, there is a need to recognize the ongoing nature of PTSD. Means of ongoing systematic emotional support should be put in place. Commissions must be created to analyze and publicly report root causes of misinformation and missteps to plan for improvements in processes during crises. As a society, we also need to express gratitude for our health and create rituals that bring us together to restore wholeness and unity in our organization and communities.

Dianne McCallister, MD, MBA
President
Diagnosis Well, Inc.

Endnotes

1. McCallister DE, Hamilton T. *Transforming the Heart of Practice: An Organizational and Personal Approach to Physician Well-being.* Cham: Springer Nature; 2019.

2. Fadel L. Doctors Say Hospitals are Stopping Them from Wearing Masks. *NPR.* 2020. https://www.npr.org/2020/04/02/825200206/doctors-say-hospitals-are-stopping-them-from-wearing-masks. Published April 2, 2020.

3. Carville O, Court E, Brown KV, Bloomberg. Hospitals Tell Doctors They'll Be Fired if They Speak Out About Lack of Gear. *Fortune.* 2020. https://fortune.com/2020/03/31/coronavirus-shortages-hospitals-doctors-fired-face-masks-ppe/. Published March 31, 2020.

4. Salber P. Healthcare Workers Say They'll Be Fired if They Wear Their Own PPE. thedoctorweighsin.com. https://thedoctorweighsin.com/healthcare-workers-ppe/. Updated April 1, 2020. Accessed.

5. Stone W, Fadel L. 'It's Like Walking Into Chernobyl,' One Doctor Says of Her Emergency Room. *NPR.* 2020. https://www.npr.org/2020/04/09/830143490/it-s-like-walking-into-chernobyl-one-doctor-says-of-her-emergency-room. Published April 9, 2020.

6. McCallister DE, Chari RS. How Physicians are Wired. In: *Transforming the Heart of Practice: An Organizational and Personal Approach to Physician Well-being.* Cham: Springer Nature; 2019.

7. Greek Medicine: The Hippocratic Oath. nlm.nih.gov. https://www.nlm.nih.gov/hmd/greek/greek_oath.html. Updated Feb. 7, 2012. Accessed.

8. Bebinger M. Threatened For Wearing a Mask or Asking for More PPE? Here are Your Legal Protections. *WBUR*. 2020. https://www.wbur.org/ commonhealth/2020/04/20/legal-protections-complaints-health-care-workers-personal-protective-equipment. Published April 20, 2020.

9. OSHA. Closed Federal and State Plan Valid Covid-19 Complaints Through May 10 Receipt Date. In: OSHA.gov, ed2020.

10. Babb K, Shammas B, Cha AE. Fallen on the Front Lines: Hundreds of Health-Care Workers Lost Their Lives Battling the Coronavirus. *The Washington Post.* 2020. https://www.washingtonpost.com/graphics/2020/health/ healthcare-workers-death-coronavirus/. Published June 17, 2020.

11. Bailey SR. Now's The Time to Have a Difficult Talk About Physician Suicide. *AMA.* 2020. https://www.ama-assn.org/about/leadership/now-s-time-have-difficult-talk-about-physician-suicide. Published Sept. 16, 2020.

12. Firth S. Could COVID-19 Pandemic Increase Physician Burnout, Suicide? *MedPage Today.* 2020. https://www.medpagetoday.com/psychiatry/ generalpsychiatry/88686. Published Sept. 17, 2020.

13. Gulati G, Kelly BD. Physician Suicide and the COVID-19 Pandemic. *Occupational Medicine.* 2020;70(7):514. doi:10.1093/occmed/kqaa104. Published June 4, 2020.

14. Arespacochaga E. Shining a Light on Physician Suicide. *American Hospital Association.* 2020. https://www.aha.org/news/blog/2020-09-17-shining-light-physician-suicide. Published Sept. 17, 2020.

15. Stern AM, Cetron MS, Markel H. The 1918–1919 Influenza Pandemic in the United States: Lessons Learned and Challenges Exposed. *Public Health Reports.* 2010;125(3_suppl):6-8.

CHAPTER 12

GRADUATE MEDICAL EDUCATION: IN PURSUIT OF WELL-BEING

Hobart Lee, MD, FAAFP
Jessica ChenFeng, PhD, LMFT
Katherine Lundrigan, MBA, CTAGME

Introduction

Graduate medical education (GME) lies in a unique place in a physician's career. It is the bridge between being a student and independent practice. Medical school, or undergraduate medical education (UME), closely resembles traditional graduate school education. Large lecture halls, textbooks, and frequent standardized tests are hallmarks of this period. Even during clerkship rotations, attendings' evaluations and standardized subject exams become the emphasis, with medical students aiming for an honors grade. The United States Medical Licensing Exam (USMLE) and Comprehensive Osteopathic Medical Licensing Exam (COMLEX) are viewed as the culmination of knowledge acquisition, a requirement to pass in order to graduate medical school, and also the National Residency Matching Program (NRMP) match into a residency program.

In contrast, physicians who have graduated from residency and fellowship are viewed largely as independent practitioners.

The American Board of Medical Specialties and their member boards require an initial board exam along with an oral board, depending on the specialty. Maintenance of certification and recertification requires continuing medical education (CME) and a recertification process with an interval exam, usually every six to ten years. The recertification process and exam often represent the floor of medical knowledge and patient safety, rather than a comprehensive evaluation and feedback for continuous improvement.

Residency and GME are the bridge between these two stages. GME transitions medical students who are used to evaluation and testing monthly to independent practice, where their recertification becomes lengthened over years. GME trains residents to move from external assessments by test grades and faculty evaluations to a more internal assessment focused on practice-based learning and self-evaluation to close knowledge gaps, improve patient care, and engage in a professional society of medicine.

Accreditation

The Accreditation Council of Graduate Medical Education (ACGME) "accredits Sponsoring Institutions and residency and fellowship programs, confers recognition on additional program formats or components, and dedicates resources to initiatives addressing areas of import in graduate medical education."[1] In 2017, ACGME updated its common program requirements, including section VI on the learning and clinical environment. Specifically, they included a section on well-being and state, "psychological, emotional, and physical well-being are critical in the development of the competent, caring, and resilient physician and require proactive attention to life inside and outside of medicine. Well-being requires that physicians retain the joy in medicine while managing their own real-life stresses . . . Residents and faculty members are at risk for burnout and depression. Programs, in partnership with their Sponsoring Institutions, have the same responsibility to address well-being as they do to ensure other aspects of resident competence . . . A positive culture in a clinical learning environment models constructive behaviors, and prepares residents with the skills and attitudes needed to thrive throughout their careers."[2]

ACGME has launched several initiatives to help address well-being for residents. The Clinical Learning Environment Review (CLER) program conducts a site visit from the ACGME to ensure compliance from sponsoring institutions. In 2017, ACGME added well-being as one of the seven items to be addressed during a site visit. In the 2020 CLER pathways to excellence, six pathways exist that focus on well-being, including topics like psychological safety, education, recognition, monitoring of workload and fatigue, resiliency training, addressing mental health and self-harm, and the systematic and institutional promotion of the physical and emotional well-being of residents.[3] ACGME's Back to Bedside project funds resident projects focused on the joy and meaning of medicine. In the first round of submission, over 200 applications were submitted, underscoring the felt need of residency programs around the country. Finally, ACGME has partnered with over 200 organizations for the National Academy of Medicine Action Collaborative on Clinician Well-Being and Resilience. Their four-year goals include:

1. Raising the visibility of clinician anxiety, burnout, depression, stress, and suicide
2. Improving baseline understanding of challenges to clinician well-being

3. Advancing evidence-based, multidisciplinary solutions to improve patient care by caring for the caregiver[4]

Journal of Graduate Medical Education

The *Journal of Graduate Medical Education* (JGME) is a journal published by ACGME focused on graduate medical education. A search of resident well-being articles shows the progress and emphasis made in addressing well-being. From 2010 to 2012, only one article was published each year that focused on resident wellness. In contrast, in 2018, 16 articles were published on resident well-being. Some of the recent articles highlight the variety of research being conducted: "Caring for the Survivors When a Resident or Fellow Dies," "In Defense of Family Leave in Surgical Residency" and "Wellness Opportunities: Sometimes It Is 'Just Time Off.'" These articles indicate the changing nature of resident well-being. Gone are the days of Q2 calls, 90+ hours per week, and the stark realization that repeated, significant, and disruptive sacrifices would need to be made to one's personal and family life in order to excel and survive residency. With the 80-hour workweek and focus on resident well-being, new challenges have emerged regarding increased team communication, the reliance on shift work, and the increased electronic health record (EHR) documentation requirements. The focus on work-life balance in the millennial generation highlights the shifting culture. The following paragraphs outline examples of what we have done in our institution as well as one example residency program to address the organizational culture and increase our focus on resident well-being.

Institutional Leadership and Vision

Supporting the well-being of residents requires institutional leadership, vision, and collaboration between our hospital leadership, the GME office, and residency program directors. At Loma Linda University Health (LLUH), one of our foundational institutional values is caring for the whole person; this is not only for the holistic (physical, psychological, social, spiritual) care of our patients, but just as importantly, for our employees and colleagues. The leadership has long recognized the importance of supporting physician well-being and established the Office of Physician Vitality (OPV) over a decade ago. Since then, we have had the opportunity to expand and develop programs for physician well-being across the system. These initiatives are described below.

Institutional Collaboration

We have on average 750 residents and fellows serving across over 40 different residency and fellowship programs. These trainees represent a significant portion of our physician workforce, and thus understanding, planning for, and responding to their well-being needs requires system-wide collaboration.

Open and Responsive Structural Support

The associate dean of our GME office continually advocates for residents' well-being. The GME administers the annual ACGME survey assessing residents' well-being, and this information is promptly shared with those who care for residents' well-being (OPV, wellness director, program directors) so that all parties can be adaptive and responsive to the expressed needs of the residents. In 2018, the associate dean established a GME position for wellness director, and one of our attending physicians now serves in this capacity. In the last two years, she has gathered a group of chief wellness residents (at least one from each program) and runs regular workshops to train (e.g., how to recognize burnout in residents, what to do when a resident has suicidal ideation, when to connect residents to professional clinical support) and update them on resources available to residents.

The wellness director is also present at the monthly GME resident forum, a one-hour space where any resident can share their concerns, offer ideas, and hear updates on resident well-being initiatives. The GME office takes all residents' concerns seriously, and one recent outcome of this listening space was the establishment of the resident concierge line to support the physical health needs of residents and their family members. Residents have direct access to the Department of Family Medicine's nurse managers who assist residents and their families in priority access to primary care services.

The OPV employs two doctoral-level licensed marriage and family therapists who offer on-call mental health services to all residents and their families. They interface regularly with programs to offer grand rounds related to physician well-being. Recent lecture topics include: "Resilience Strategies and Burnout Prevention," "Managing Sleep Deprivation and Fatigue," "Physician Depression and Suicide," "Building Day-to-Day Brain Resilience," "Creating Safe and Equitable Working Environments" and "Navigating Perfectionism with Self-Compassion." They also meet regularly with the GME wellness director to discuss issues and update plans relevant to resident well-being. Because of the strong relationships that the OPV has established with the program directors, directors often reach out to the OPV regarding residents who are struggling or need connection to services.

Responding to 2020

The events of 2020 have tested the responsiveness and collaborative partnerships of LLUH's institutional systems. As soon as the COVID-19 pandemic began, our GME associate dean immediately established a semiweekly call to update residents on the status of COVID-19, including access to personal protective equipment in our hospitals, and respond to any concerns and questions. In this space, leadership could hear the on-the-ground concerns of residents (e.g., childcare issues, time-off protocols while COVID-19 test results were pending, PPE protocols, etc.) and troubleshoot ways to establish policies that would better support them.

All residency programs immediately shifted to virtual meetings and found innovative ways to keep residents socially connected and supported through safe, socially distanced gatherings or creatively utilizing their social media platforms to connect residents to one another.

The GME office also recognized how the increased racial injustice and uprisings in 2020 would impact residents and hosted a virtual event "Coming Together for #Blacklivesmatter." At this event, representatives across the campus (chaplains, mental health clinicians, diversity and equity advocates) were present to offer thoughtful reflections, provide support, and give residents opportunity to respond as a community. Subsequently, campus diversity, equity, and inclusion initiatives have expanded with many residents taking the lead.

Residents' Knowledge Of and Access To Support

There are several avenues through which our residents learn about and can access support for their wellness. After the results of the NRMP match, our GME office emails newly matched residents to provide information for all our wellness resources and encourages them to make appointments. The GME office also reaches out to residents with unusual circumstances during UME or previous GME training to ensure that they start off their training with as much support as needed, including connecting them to a therapist, psychiatrist, or other support. In 2020, we also reached out to incoming residents and fellows from national COVID-19 hotspots to offer them clinical support in case of PTSD or other COVID-19-related stress.

Once residents have arrived at LLUH, they get a chance to meet members of the wellness team at orientation and are given contact information for:

- ⊙ Office of Physician Vitality (OPV)
- ⊙ Employee Assistance Program (EAP): cost-free, short-term therapy for residents and their families
- ⊙ Community Mental Health Providers: insurance-covered therapy options with clinicians in the community
- ⊙ Faculty Psychiatrist: direct access to a psychiatrist without a referral
- ⊙ Physician Well-Being Committee: confidential support for physicians with substance abuse
- ⊙ Primary Care Priority Access Line: direct access to a nurse manager in Family Medicine to help facilitate appointments and access to services

Throughout their training, residents are continually reminded of the resources available to them through grand rounds, their chief wellness residents, the GME resident forum, and a monthly resident e-newsletter. Programs are scheduling wellness days for their residents, which include a time to meet with the OPV clinicians for a "wellness check" and confidentially discuss their well-being.

Family Medicine Residency

From a Family Medicine residency standpoint, we applied the overarching LLUH institutional policies to our individual program level to impact resident well-being. We take a multipronged approach to ensure our culture keeps our residents resilient, engaged, and well from match day all the way through graduation. This involves adding our own residency "support" pillars upon LLUH's strong foundation to build a sense of family within the program itself. We take steps to support our core teaching faculty, who we see as our attending physician role models, as well as steps to support residents directly.

Family Medicine Core Teaching Faculty Support

The Department of Family Medicine considers our core teaching faculty to be the primary group of physician educators who are driven to create an excellent residency learning experience. Ensuring these individuals are resilient, engaged, and well is the first step in ensuring the desired positive culture is being modeled to our residents. This meets our ACGME requirements but also enables greater satisfaction as reported by residents, faculty, and staff; reduces burnout and turnover in our clinics; and ultimately provides a better experience for our patients.

Faculty schedules are prioritized so that all core teaching faculty can come together each month to discuss programmatic and individual resident progress. Additionally, periodic retreats are held for core teaching faculty for purposes of comradery, faculty development, and programmatic improvement. Off-campus retreats bring a fresh opportunity for us to feel creative and play games, such as those designed to specifically improve leadership competencies. This helps us feel more connected to our purpose and allows us to formulate goals for the program that are both achievable and inspiring. We combine our Annual Program Evaluation (APE) day with our annual residency retreat, where core teaching faculty, residents, and staff can come together in both fellowship and work.

Annually, we assess for burnout in our core teaching faculty, staff, and residents. The data from this inventory is tracked over time and is used to measure the overall program burnout level. Individual resident data is confidentially reviewed by a psychologist. Those individuals who have been identified as "at risk" are provided a list of resources available for optional use (including the OPV) and encouraged to seek ways to increase their personal wellness.

With the aim of preventing burnout in both resident and core teaching faculty, a group consisting of faculty and staff participated in the Institute for Healthcare Improvement's (IHI) 12-week online course with coaching entitled, "Finding and Creating Joy in Work."[5] This group defined joy as "more than the absence of burnout" and focused on improving faculty and staff collegiality and relationships.

As core teaching faculty model how to practice medicine, they also model cultural norms and behaviors, and set expectations for our residents. We believe when the core teaching faculty are resilient, engaged, and well, the program and residents benefit. To this end, the Department of Family Medicine has engaged in flexible scheduling and fair compensation models for the core teaching faculty.

Family Medicine Resident Support

Our resident support begins on match day as the program director congratulates and welcomes our new, incoming interns. The administrative staff begin the process of onboarding, and our current residents connect with these incoming interns, helping them feel a part of our community. Incoming interns are assigned a faculty advisor and a resident "big sibling," both of whom become supportive resources throughout a resident's training.

Residents who join our residency program are starting both a new job and a new educational training period. As employees, they have employment contracts, and as trainees, they have educational competencies they must achieve. To best prepare our incoming interns to be outstanding and well residents, we devote the first four weeks of their residency to an extended orientation. They are given overviews on policies and procedures as well as time to adjust to their new responsibilities. Interspersed throughout orientation is specific time to bond as a cohort, learn more about themselves as individuals, and engage in the wellness benefits available to them. One practical example is that our program schedules each new intern to meet with EAP, even prior to any concerns about stress or burnout. This appointment gives each new intern the opportunity to participate in the process and lowers the psychological barriers to care before problems arise, creating a culture where seeking help is encouraged and celebrated rather than viewed as a character weakness or moral failing.

The program encourages resident social events. Elected resident "social chairs" plan and oversee activities that include such things as weddings and baby showers, holiday parties, and community service events. "Resident support groups" are held monthly so residents can debrief together, practice techniques like mindfulness, and are moderated by the OPV or outside faculty.

Monthly, we ask faculty, residents, or staff to share about themselves both in- and outside of the program—details like why they chose this specialty, who their support people are, how they define and engage in spirituality, and what they like to do to relax. We call this presentation, "About me," and it offers a personal connection before we engage in our monthly resident admin meeting.

The Family Medicine residency program strives to meet both the needs of our patients while recognizing the needs of the individual residents themselves. We know our residents have relationships, hobbies, and other personal needs outside of their programmatic responsibilities that can contribute significant noncognitive stress affecting their performance and ultimately patient care. By offering flexible scheduling and allowing incoming interns to pick a block rotation "track," we give incoming interns autonomy and agency to pick a schedule, including vacation times, that works best for them.

Conclusion

GME represents the crucial fundamental training period for physicians. The accelerated learning in both medical knowledge and patient care remain challenging, but in hindsight, the professional role models and friendships that form remain seminal to the understanding of what it means to be a "physician" and a contributing member in our community and society at large. As GME occurs in this critical developmental period of professional identity, we remain hopeful that a focus on well-being during residency will create another generation of physicians who engage in whole-person care for their patients as well as for themselves.

Thanks

We would like to thank Dr. Roger Woodruff and Dr. Daniel Giang for their support and commitment to residency well-being and education.

Hobart Lee, MD, FAAFP
Associate Professor, Department of Family Medicine
Director, Family Medicine Residency Program
Loma Linda University Health

Jessica ChenFeng, PhD, LMFT
Associate Professor of Medical Education
Associate Director of Physician Vitality
Loma Linda University Health

Katherine Lundrigan, MBA, CTAGME
Associate Program Director
Family Medicine Residency Program
Loma Linda University Health

Endnotes

1. What We Do. ACGME. https://www.acgme.org/What-We-Do/Overview. Published 2020. Accessed 2020-10-07.

2. ACGME. Common Program Requirements. https://www.acgme.org/Portals/0/PFAssets/ProgramRequirements/CPRResidency2020_TCC.pdf. Published 2020. Accessed 2020-10-07.

3. Organization ACfGM. *CLER Pathways to Excellence: Expectations for an Optimal Clinical Learning Environment to Achieve Safe and High-Quality Patient Care, version 2.0.* Chicago, IL: Accreditation Council for Graduate Medical Education; 2019.

4. NAoM. Action Collaborative on Clinician Well-Being and Resilience. https://nam.edu/initiatives/clinician-resilience-and-well-being/. Published 2020. Accessed 2020-10-07.

5. Perlo J, Balik B, Swensen S, Kabcenell A, Landsman J, Feeley D. IHI Framework for Improving Joy in Work [IHI White Paper]. *Institute for Healthcare Improvement.* 2017.

CHAPTER 13

RELATIONSHIP-CENTERED COMMUNICATION: WILL AND SKILL

Pam Guler, MHA, FACHE
Calvin Chou, MD, PhD

Introduction

"Dr. Sampson is one of the most caring physicians I have ever had. You never feel like she is rushing to get you out the door, and she seems genuinely concerned for your health and any questions you might have. She was a godsend during a very scary and difficult time. I would absolutely refer her to anybody and everybody I can."

"Dr. Daniel is very kind, concerned, and articulate in explaining concerns and coming up with a plan of treatment that is reasonable, while also taking into consideration my emotional well-being. He is the kind of doctor that inspires confidence and makes me feel comfortable about expressing concerns and asking questions."

TRUST . . . a crucial concept that can and should weave through the DNA of a patient-provider relationship. Imagine for a moment if every person felt the level of trust seen in these real patients' remarks about their physicians and the impact this could have on health outcomes and care experience. Then, imagine how these physicians feel when and after interacting with these patients. In the following pages, we'll explore the impact of relationship-centered communication between physicians and their patients: why relationships matter and what exactly comprises this method of communicating. We'll also explore the cultural impact that an organization can achieve when all who serve within it communicate effectively with empathy.

The Impact of Relationship-Centered Communication on Patients

We estimate that physicians have more than 200,000 face-to-face (or virtual) patient interactions during their careers. This number does not include telephone calls or secure messaging with patients and their families, nor the innumerable meetings and conversations they enter into with colleagues and interdisciplinary teams. Yet, until relatively recently, most physicians received little or no formal training in what we see as the most common procedure that all perform: communication! Would you trust a surgeon who admitted that they had received little formal training, observed few experts, received scant feedback, and determined their methods only by trial and error for a procedure they were going to perform on you?

In addition, the way that physicians optimally communicate with patients and, indeed, the way that patients are beginning to expect their physicians to interact with them, emphasizes two-way communication and understanding, rather than a unidirectional download. This approach to care is one important facet of relationship-centered care which focuses on the space between health care clinicians (along with their teams) and patients (along with the families and systems that support them) and how each bring themselves and their emotions to the conversation. When we emphasize the relationship rather than an individual, we can obtain a broader understanding of the important influences on a patient's care.

Impact on Patient Health Outcomes

Effective relationship-centered communication leads to better outcomes for patients. Intuitively, we recognize that effective communication improves understanding of a plan of care and the potential for patient adherence to that plan, ultimately impacting outcomes and overall health status. Studies have also shown that effective communication leads to better outcomes in specific diseases and chronic illness, including, for example with cancer patients, increased adherence to cancer screening,[1] better care at end of life, and improved length of survival.[2] Patients of physicians with high empathy scores, measured by a validated scale, were significantly more likely to have good control of diabetes and cholesterol.[3] Mortality from myocardial infarction decreases because of effective communication with patients.[4] Post-surgical outcomes are improved by effective communication. The incidence of serious postoperative outcomes, such as cardiac arrhythmia[5] and delirium,[6] decreases. Patients who perceived their trauma surgeon as being more empathic had better medical outcomes after hospitalization.[7]

Impact on Patient Experience of Care

Effective communication also leads to enhanced patient experience of care. Of course, the ultimate measure of patient experience with their physician is seen in the trust that develops between the two and the impact on patient well-being and health outcomes. There are national measures of patient experience as well. One such measure is seen via the Consumer Assessment of Healthcare Providers and Systems (CAHPS) family of the Center for Medicare and Medicaid Services (CMS) surveys, such as Hospital Consumer Assessment of Healthcare Providers and Systems (HCAHPS) in the hospital inpatient setting or the Clinical and Group Consumer Assessment of Healthcare Providers and Systems (CG-CAHPS) in a clinician and group practice setting.

Questions around communication on these surveys do not measure only "satisfaction" but also ask about the frequency that specific types of communication happen during an encounter. These surveys also explicitly ask whether physicians listened to their patient, treated them with courtesy and respect, and explained things to them in a way they could understand. A national health system study showed that relationship-centered communication training and intentional application of the concepts had a stronger impact on particularly the HCAHPS doctor communication question regarding courtesy and respect. The same study showed that with the introduction of a relationship-centered approach to communication, doctor communication ratings in the physician practice setting statistically improved across the board.[8] A national review of comments about physicians on these surveys showed that patients repeatedly note how important it is for them to perceive that their physician and staff show that they care. The clearest way of showing caring is through intentional and effective communication.[9] In fact, additional questions asked on AdventHealth inpatient surveys indicate that four of the most highly correlated topics to an overall excellent experience include: the physician kept you informed; the physician showed concern for your questions/worries; the staff worked together to care for you; and the staff addressed emotional needs. These topics form the core of relationship-centered communication both between the care team and patient and within the care team themselves.

Unfortunately, literature shows that clinicians do not always communicate as effectively as they think. Certainly, systemic factors interfere with the way that most clinicians would like to practice optimally. Even so, a gap exists between what physicians think they're doing and what they're actually doing.

Studies have shown that physicians tend to interrupt within 11 seconds of a patient beginning to speak.[10] Physicians and other clinicians often use jargon and acronyms that are not understandable to patients. The impact of poor communication can be seen in a lack of patient loyalty, readmissions, and malpractice claims.

The Impact of Relationship-Centered Communication on Physicians

"To me the greatest aspect of being a physician is the relationship you get to form with patients who trust you to know every aspect of their lives. The patient actually is willing to put their life in my hands and trusts that I have the needed knowledge to recommend to them all of their treatment options. These relationships usually go much deeper than the physical and emotional, as the opportunity to address their spiritual needs through conversation and prayer often present themselves."

Physicians who intentionally leverage relationship-centered communication techniques achieve benefits well beyond patient experience results. All physicians at some point have challenges and difficult conversations in their practice that can leave them feeling unsettled and dissatisfied. Learning to communicate more effectively with patients helps physicians not only make more accurate diagnoses and enhance adherence to treatment but also increases their own well-being and resilience.[9] Several studies at different health systems corroborate this important finding. Clinicians who participated in a mindful communication program had higher well-being and attitudes toward patient care.[11] Clinicians who underwent a daylong communication skills course showed increased empathy scores and lower burnout scores when compared with those who did not.[9]

"The most surprising thing that's happened over and over during my years of practice is that I've formed the closest of bonds with my patients who have gone through challenges and tragedies. Patients that I've learned from the most and have imprinted on me forever are those who have lost a baby, those who have had to work through complications, and certainly those who have been through abuse or assault. Getting close to them and their families has shaped me as a physician and as a person. We cannot be whole without feeling pain, and we cannot achieve our personal best without struggles. Living those patients' struggles and hurt with them molds me into the physician that I always want to be."

The How of Relationship-Centered Communication

Our goal within this section is to provide an overview of the key components of relationship-centered communication for physicians. More expansive books related to the step-by-step skill sets and practices are readily available—in particular, publications from the Academy of Communication in Healthcare, such as *Communication Rx*.[9]

Relationship-centered communication has at its core in the concepts of listening, empathy, and efficient agenda-setting for patient-physician interactions. We list the specific skill sets in the following table.

SKILL SET ONE: BEGINNING THE ENCOUNTER
Open with a warm greeting and attend to comfort
Acknowledge communication barriers (e.g., computer)
Elicit the list of all concerns
Negotiate an agenda for the time to be spent in this encounter

SKILL SET TWO: SKILLS THAT BUILD TRUST
Ask open-ended questions and listen actively
Elicit patient's ideas and expectations
Name the patient's emotions and respond with empathys
Transition to further data gathering/medical exam

SKILL SET THREE: DELIVERING DIAGNOSES AND TREATMENT PLANS
Collaborate on a plan that the patient can follow
Leverage teach-back to ensure proper two-way transmission

Table 1: Relationship-Centered Communication Skill Sets[9]

In a nutshell, these skill sets allow the physician to be meaningfully present with the patient and explore their needs more fully. We'll discuss some important features of these skill sets in order.

Skill Set 1: Beginning the Encounter

From the very beginning, investing in a positive first impression situates an encounter to succeed. This investment starts before an encounter, when physicians can take a moment to center themselves in the present, quickly metabolizing emotional residue from previous encounters and tasks that may unduly influence the patient at hand. A warm greeting and "small talk before big talk" may help grease the wheels before getting down to business. Although Skill Set 1 may appear to lengthen patient-physician interactions with the approach of eliciting the full list of concerns, in reality, getting all items in the open at the outset of the visit reduces the number of "door-knob questions" that may be critically important. It can be very frustrating for physicians to feel they are nearing the end of a visit, only to encounter a last-minute item such as, "Oh, by the way, I have chest pain." Finally, negotiating an agenda for the visit allows both patient and physician to collaboratively determine the priorities for the encounter, again placing emphasis on relationship formation.

Skill Set 2: Skills That Build Trust

In Skill Set 2, remaining in the present moment pertains to the entire encounter as well: active listening is key to reinforcing the basis of trust in the entire interaction. This is much more easily said than done because physicians often think distractedly about differential diagnosis, medication refills, and sometimes more tangential topics while patients are talking. Instead, it is important to concentrate on both the content and emotion of what patients say. Responding to their emotion in empathetic ways is key to showing that we care.

There are two kinds of responses, both of which are valuable and both of which depend on the fact that physicians need to listen closely. The first kind of response is to summarize the content of what we heard. For patients, hearing their words repeated back can help them feel that the physician has been listening. For physicians, talking through what patients have said can clarify facts as well as the clinical reasoning process. The second kind of response, responding to emotions, takes a little more effort. Patients rarely intersect with physicians without some kind of emotion, so naming their emotion and using empathic statements can help patients feel even more that their physician is truly listening.

Skill Set 3: Delivering Diagnoses and Treatment Plans

Skill Set 3 involves sharing information and asking for a teach-back. At times, physicians get frustrated when patients don't do what they tell them to do. This may ultimately be the fault of the physician, who may have downloaded a lot of information, including jargon and acronyms. Even if the physician asks, "Do you have any questions?" at the end of an encounter, patients may be too polite—or overwhelmed—to ask. Having the patient "teach back" or share with the physician their understanding of what has been discussed is an excellent way of ensuring understanding and ultimate adherence to the plan of care. Though this process can feel awkward, a physician can orient patients by saying, for example, "I know I spoke a lot just now. Just so I know I made myself clear, tell me what you will do when you go home."

The Skill Sets and Virtual Visits

With the conversion to largely virtual visits in the pandemic era, the importance of relationship-centered communication remains high. Though the usual elements of in-person interactions have been disrupted, the necessity of developing and maintaining these professional relationships persists. Fortunately, all of the above skill sets apply very well to virtual encounters, with minor adaptations: (1) addressing communication barriers now involves explicit questions about our ability to hear (and see, for video visits) each other and about who else might be in earshot or out of view, and (2) with decreased ability to interpret nonverbal cues, due to the virtual medium and/or the use of personal protective equipment, asking explicitly about emotion and demonstrating verbal empathy hold even weightier impact.

Cultural Impact

We have thus far mainly focused on relationship-centered communication in the patient-physician pair. It is not a leap to consider how these same principles, adapted to all conversations in health care (between physician and family members, between interprofessional members of the care team and the patient, among interprofessional colleagues, between frontline care delivery personnel and administrative leadership, and on and on), is critical to establishing a culture of whole-person care. Above, we referenced the salutary effect that training in relationship-centered communication can have on individual physicians' burnout and resilience. From a systems-level perspective, these skill sets are intertwined with individual and external factors that the National Academy of Medicine has determined exert influence on well-being and resilience at both personal and institutional levels.[12] Imagine the impact on a health care system if all members of the team communicated effectively, truly listened, showed empathy to one another, and ensured that an explanation or, in the case of patients, a treatment plan was fully understood. A holistic focus on mind, body, and spirit for all involved could be achieved.

Conclusion

"As a physician we often ask people to bare their souls; to tell us things that they may not have told anyone else. More so, we ask them to do that within just a few minutes of meeting them. I hold this trust I am given with the utmost care. I hope that I create a safe place where people can come and truly get the help and guidance that they need."

TRUST . . . a word that started this chapter and a word that will close it. The trust between physician and patient is a sacred bond. Nothing instills trust more than the feeling that another person knows you, cares about you, listens to you, and has the expertise to guide you to a best outcome. Communicating in a relationship-centered manner takes practice and intention and has the power to connect in ways that improve quality, safety, and experience, helping both ourselves and those we serve to feel whole.

Pam Guler, MHA, FACHE
Vice President and Chief Experience Officer
AdventHealth

Calvin Chou, MD, PhD
Professor of Clinical Medicine
University of California at San Francisco

Endnotes

1. Fox SA, Heritage J, Stockdale SE, Asch SM, Duan N, Reise SP. Cancer screening adherence: Does physician–patient communication matter? *Patient Education and Counseling.* 2009;75(2):178-184.

2. Temel JS, Greer JA, Muzikansky A, et al. Early palliative care for patients with metastatic non-small-cell lung cancer. *New England Journal of Medicine.* 2010;363(8):733-742.

3. Hojat M, Louis D, Markham F, Wender R, Rabinowitz C, Gonnella J. Physicians' empathy and clinical outcomes for diabetic patients. *Academic Medicine: Journal of the Association of American Medical Colleges.* 2011;86(3):359-364.

4. Meterko M, Wright S, Lin H, Lowy E, Cleary PD. Mortality among Patients with Acute Myocardial Infarction: The Influences of Patient-Centered Care and Evidence-Based Medicine. *Health Services Research.* 2010;45(5p1):1188-1204.

5. Trummer U, Mueller U, Nowak P, Stidl T, Pelikan J. Does physician-patient communication that aims at empowering patients improve clinical outcome? A case study. *Patient Education and Counseling.* 2006;61(2):299-306.

6. Lee J, Jung J, Noh JS, Yoo S, Hong YS. Perioperative Psycho-Educational Intervention Can Reduce Postoperative Delirium in Patients after Cardiac Surgery: A Pilot Study. *The International Journal of Psychiatry in Medicine.* 2013;45(2):143-158.

7. Steinhausen S, Ommen O, Antoine S-L, Koehler T, Pfaff H, Neugebauer E. Short- and long-term subjective medical treatment outcome of trauma surgery patients: the importance of physician empathy. *Patient Preference and Adherence.* 2014;8:1239-1253.

8. Boissy A, Windover AK, Bokar D, et al. Communication Skills Training for Physicians Improves Patient Satisfaction. *Journal of General Internal Medicine.* 2016;31(7):755-761.

9. Chou C, Cooley L. *Communication Rx: Transforming Healthcare through Relationship-Centered Communication.* United States: McGraw-Hill Education; 2018.

10. Singh Ospina N, Phillips KA, Rodriguez-Gutierrez R, et al. Eliciting the Patient's Agenda- Secondary Analysis of Recorded Clinical Encounters. *Journal of General Internal Medicine.* 2019;34(1):36-40.

11. Krasner MS, Epstein RM, Beckman H, et al. Association of an Educational Program in Mindful Communication With Burnout, Empathy, and Attitudes Among Primary Care Physicians. *JAMA.* 2009;302(12):1284-1293.

12. Education ACfGM, Nurses AAoCC, Pharmacists ASoHS, et al. A Journey to Construct an All-Encompassing Conceptual Model of Factors Affecting Clinician Well-Being and Resilience. *NAM Perspectives.* 2018;8(1).

CHAPTER 14

FINDING MEANING IN MEDICINE: A STORYTELLING GROUP EXPERIENCE

J. Michael Yurso, MD, FACS
Burt Bertram, EdD, LMHC

Introduction

Core to work satisfaction is the extent to which work contributes to a meaningful life. The Finding Meaning in Medicine® (FMM) storytelling group experience described below was developed by Rachel Remen, MD. This chapter is based on the authors' seven-year collaboration where they established and conducted a Finding Meaning in Medicine group at a midsize hospital within the AdventHealth System. The chapter begins with a brief overview of the sources of the meaning of work and the mechanics of how work becomes meaningful. Readers are provided a "how to" for establishing a Finding Meaning in Medicine group in their hospital that includes the history, philosophy, organization, structure, and flow of the experience. The authors conclude the chapter with an insider's look at their experience of facilitating the group and a perspective on the impact the group had on the more than 60 physicians who participated in one or more meetings.

Meaningfulness of Work

The dynamics associated with meaning in work or what is often referred to by scholars as the "meaningfulness of work"[1] have been investigated for many years, resulting in a substantial reservoir of data. Authors Rosso, Dekas, and Wrzesniewski conducted an extensive review of the meaning of work literature and concluded that there are two broad areas of influence associated with the study of the meaningfulness of work: (1) the sources of the meaning of work, and (2) how work becomes meaningful.[2]

Sources of the Meaning of Work

The Self includes the values, the motivations, and the beliefs about the purpose of work. Beliefs govern the "degree of congruence between one's needs and perceptions that the job can meet those needs. The more involved one is with the job, the more difficult it is to dissociate oneself or one's self-esteem from that job, making that work more meaningful."[3] Work orientation beliefs are also an important factor. Is work a job (means to financial end), a career (focus on advancement, pay, and prestige within an organization), or does work emerge from an internal beckoning, what some would refer to as a "calling," that is associated with the belief that the work contributes to a greater good and makes the world a better place? Callings can be "secular," in which work is an expression of a person's deepest self, or "sacred," which imbues work with both meaning and meaningfulness through the sense that one is serving God and meeting the needs of the larger community.

Others involves how an individual's interactions and relationships with other persons or groups, both within and outside the workplace, influence the meaning of work. The most obvious example of this is how "others" within the organization (coworkers, colleagues, supervisors, etc.) express/demonstrate awareness of the value or contribution of an individual and her/his role or performance. Others can also extend outside of the organization to include positive (or negative) expressions by family or friends about a person's work.

The Context in which work occurs is another important source of work meaning. Context in this regard is an extremely broad collection of influences[4] that includes the significance of the tasks involved in the job, the mission/purpose of the organization, monetary rewards and how work enhances/detracts from important nonwork domains of life (family, hobbies, recreation and work-life balance).

Spiritual Life is an area of ongoing research. Some studies have found that an individual's religion can play an important role in how they conduct their work lives. Spiritual life can serve to connect the ego to something greater than oneself and/or work can be experienced as a sacred calling through which God's will is done. Research shows that spiritual employees perceive their work differently than nonspiritual employees, seeing their work behaviors in spiritual terms of caring service and transcendence. Therefore, when employees perceive work in a spiritual light, their work is likely to take on a deeper sense of meaningfulness and purpose for them.[5]

How Work Becomes Meaningful

Researchers have identified seven psychological and social "mechanisms"[6] that invite or facilitate the meaningfulness of work. We briefly outline these below and will return to these mechanisms when we discuss outcomes from the Finding Meaning in Medicine experience.

Authenticity—involves work that supports and promotes the authentic self, because it enables individuals to maintain consistency with valued attitudes, beliefs, values, and identities while working.[7]

Self-efficacy—the belief that a person has the power and ability to produce an intended effect or to make a difference.

Self-esteem—involves feelings of accomplishment or affirmation resulting from work experiences that help to fulfill individuals' motivation for believing they are valuable and worthy individuals.[8]

Purpose—is related to the significance of the work. A clear and higher purpose evokes a sense of duty and motivation.

Belongingness—is recognized to play a sizeable influence on an individuals' perception of the meaningfulness of work. Membership in, identification with, and feelings of connection to social groups through work may provide individuals with meaningfulness by helping them experience a positive sense of common identity, fate, or humanity with others.[9]

Transcendence—refers to connecting or superseding the ego to an entity greater than the self or beyond the material world.

Cultural and interpersonal sensemaking—work has value to the extent that the collective culture has deemed it to be valuable and/or to the prevailing interpersonal positive expressions of work colleagues.

Challenges to Meaningfulness in the Practice of Medicine Today

The challenges to meaningfulness in the practice of medicine are well documented. We refer readers to an extensive body of literature on the topic[10] that delves into the sea of changes, obstacles, and threats that confront every practicing physician, some of which include narrowing of insurance networks, financial pressures, and the resulting increase in expectations in terms of patient productivity, increased workload, and reduced physician autonomy. At the same time, physicians have been required to navigate a rapidly expanding medical knowledge base, more onerous maintenance of certifications requirements, increased clerical burden associated with electronic medical records, new regulatory requirements (meaningful use, e-prescribing, medication reconciliation), and an unprecedented level of scrutiny (quality metrics, patient satisfaction scores, measures of cost).[11]

Tait Shanafelt, MD, and associates are likely the most prolific and respected voices on the topic of physician well-being and burnout. They make the case that addressing physician burnout and well-being requires a coordinated effort at the national, state, organization, leader, and individual levels.[12] The Finding Meaning in Medicine storytelling experience is a positive action that can be taken at the organization, leader, and individual levels. To that end, what follows is a description of the origin and history of Finding Meaning in Medicine (and a report from the authors of their experience coordinating and facilitating more than 20 FMM group meetings over a seven-year period in one hospital within a large health care system.

FMM Origin and History

In 1998, Rachel Remen, MD, began a storytelling discussion group for her colleagues.[13] Dr. Remen had, for many years, been interested in and concerned about the lives and well-being of practicing physicians. As an author, speaker, and practicing physician, she had the opportunity to speak to other physicians from around the country about their lived experience as a physician. Through those encounters, she imagined a time and space when physicians could come together and talk about the deeper meaning of their work. Over the next couple of years, she conceived and piloted a group discussion experience for physicians that was built around giving physicians an opportunity to tell a story, in the company of other physicians, about their experience as a physician.

By 2000, she had written a detailed resource guide that describes the purpose, structure, and process of organizing and facilitating a Finding Meaning in Medicine discussion group for physicians.[14] Now, under the auspices of the Remen Institute for the Study of Health and Illness, Finding Meaning in Medicine discussion groups have been expanded beyond physicians to include groups for nurses,

> **Finding Meaning in Medicine** is a conversation that invites physicians to speak from the heart . . . physician-to-physician about personal experiences in their everyday life that provide access to the deeper meaning of the practice of medicine.

residents, medical students, and interprofessional/ interdisciplinary professionals. Each one-hour discussion group is built around an announced topic, generally captured by one word (e.g., "Compassion" or "Empathy" or "Listening" or "Grace") or dozens of other evocative words that conjure up a moment of interaction between a caregiver and a patient, family member, or colleague. The "price of admission" is a first-person story from the attendees. The stories are personal; they reveal the private internal person of the professional caregiver. They are heartfelt stories that generate reverent silence, smiles, tears, and sometimes even laughter as participants identify with the storyteller's experience. All the stories invite the teller of the story, as well as the listener of the story, to remember the deeper meaning of the practice of medicine. Everyone is invited but is never required to share a story.

Authors' FMM Experience: Organization & Flow

The Finding Meaning in Medicine experience at Florida Hospital Altamonte, now AdventHealth Altamonte, was initiated by Herdley Paolini, PhD, the director of physician support services and passionately supported by Rob Fulbright, CEO. She reached out to General Surgeon Mike Yurso, MD, who was the medical executive at Florida Hospital Altamonte, to solicit his interest in forming and facilitating an FMM group. As an incentive, she offered the assistance of Burt Bertram, EdD (consulting psychotherapist and experienced group facilitator). Dr. Remen's original model is conceived as physician-led and does not involve a mental health professional. While not essential, it was our experience that having co-facilitators was a great advantage, and the combination of a practicing physician and experienced group facilitator made for a powerful team.

In the beginning and throughout the seven years of the group, Dr. Yurso personally invited every physician he encountered in the halls and lounge to come to his home (three miles from the hospital) for a light dinner followed by our FMM discussion. Physicians came and returned again. Initially, there were five or six attendees, but by the end of the first year, the average attendance was 12–14 and growing. On a couple of occasions, more than 20 physicians attended. Over the course of the seven years, more than 60 physicians showed up at one or more meetings. More than 20 physicians attended eight or more meetings. Invitees are asked to RSVP; many do, some don't, and inevitably some who planned to attend are unable to, while others decide to come at the last minute. As a result of this open format, the attendee composition of each Finding Meaning in Medicine gathering is always different and, to a degree, unpredictable. The facilitators are never sure exactly who or how many participants will take part.

For each meeting, the topic was decided in advance. Most often the topic had been determined at the end of the previous meeting. Topics for our meetings included:

MEETING TOPICS		
Work/Life Balance	Compassion	Listening
Mistakes & Forgiveness	Anger	Trust
Renewal	Humility	Spirit-Spirituality-Prayer
Gratitude	Forgiveness	Service
Humor & Laughter	Collaboration	Honesty

On one occasion, we had a couples meeting where we invited physicians to bring their spouse or significant other. The topic for that evening was the Medical Marriage.

Finding Meaning in Medicine is a two-and-a-half-hour experience that typically unfolds in the following manner:

TWO-AND-A-HALF-HOUR EXPERIENCE	
6:00 – 6:45 p.m.	Dinner/Social
6:45 – 8:15 p.m.	Conversation
8:15 – 8:30 p.m.	Closure & Choice of Topic for the Next Gathering

Following the dinner and social time, the physician host and co-facilitator would begin the experience by introducing the topic for the evening. The mental health professional co-facilitator reviewed the ground rules. This review sounded something like the following:

"We begin by asking that you keep these conversations confidential. If you find this meeting beneficial and wish to tell another, we ask that you do it in such a way that would not identify the object of the story or the storyteller. We ask that you practice respectful listening; please, no interruptions. We are not here to solve problems, so please resist giving advice; we are simply here to support one another. Each of us very likely has a story that fits the topic of the evening."

It is important to begin each gathering by reminding participants of the ground rules. This ritual ensures that everyone, veterans as well as first timers, understands the expectations of the group experience.

GROUND RULES
Speak . . . when/if you are moved to do so
Be . . . as fully present as possible (step out if you need to make a call)
Listen . . . deeply, attentively, and without judgment.
Resist . . . any urge to problem-solve, give advice, or fix anything or anyone
Respect . . . confidentiality of what is said and by whom.

Facilitating group member interaction involves the careful monitoring of the process to ensure that the ground rules are observed. It is important to gently intervene if problem-solving or advice-giving breaks out, if the topic drifts into an unrelated one or away from the announced topic, or if someone is talking too much. Time management is essential to allow for everyone to have a share of airtime. Silence is another aspect of time management. When silence descends on the process, it can be anxiety-provoking for the facilitators. Two minutes of silence can feel like forever. Take a breath . . . give it a few moments; often silence is evidence of quiet self-reflection or the internal processing of what just occurred or the internal experience of preparing to speak. As the time for closure draws close, one of the facilitators generally will invite any attendees who have not yet spoken to have the opportunity to tell her/his story. Finally, it is time to choose a topic for the next meeting. Often the next topic is obvious, as it surfaced during the discussion.

At the conclusion of the evening, after all the participants had departed, we found it useful to take 15–20 minutes to review the evening with an eye toward identifying opportunities to improve the process and/or to acknowledge in-the-moment decisions that either facilitator made that enhanced or detracted from the experience. On a couple of occasions, we needed to unpack comments or actions of attendees that distracted the process and discuss how we could better prepare for or facilitate such experiences in the future.

The Impact of the Group Experience

Assessing the outcome/benefit of any group experience is layered with complexity. Voluntary attendance and participation are, of course, the best indicators that the experience is meaningful and worth the investment of time. We heard anecdotal reports of positive outcomes, including comments Dr. Yurso received from colleagues about how much they appreciated the opportunity to learn more about their physician colleagues and how that deeper understanding enhanced their collaboration. Additionally, an anonymous survey asking participants to respond to five questions was distributed in the fall of 2013. More than one half of the respondents indicated the meetings helped establish new collaborative relationships with physician colleagues and fostered mindfulness in relationships with patients. We were fortunate to have the institutional resources to create a video that told the story of our FMM gatherings. The video included comments from several attendees, one of whom offered a summation of the experience with the comment, "I come, not really looking for anything in particular, but I always leave with something that I needed."

As we reflect on these data and the in-hospital interaction between and among many of the physician attendees, we are mindful of all seven categories of "how work becomes meaningful."

Authenticity—Emotional safety in the Finding Meaning in Medicine experience was a high priority. Restating the ground rules at the beginning of every meeting underscored the importance of these guidelines and worked to create both group cohesion and a culture of emotional honesty. Authentic first-person disclosures were invited and modeled. Members dropped their professional personas, took risks, and talked vulnerably about experiences that were both sublime and frightening. Members demonstrated acceptance, respect, and support for each other, all of which invited deeper authenticity.

Self-efficacy—Throughout every meeting, as members told their stories, we could see nods and smiles from listeners who communicated "I get it" to the speaker. Whether the speaker was describing a funny interaction with a patient, relating a humbling moment of crisis in the operating room, or quietly sitting with a patient and family as they absorbed the confirmation of a diagnosis, the physician-to-physician recognition communicated a clear message: You made a difference.

Self-esteem—Self-esteem is enhanced when affirmations are heartfelt and especially powerful when expressed among peers. It was surprising how often another doctor, sometimes sitting in the room, became an important character in the story being told. These moments of gratitude confirmed the worth and value not just of the "other doctor" in the story but of all doctors everywhere.

Purpose—The belief that one's work has a higher purpose is a potent motivator to give all of oneself despite fatigue, time away from family and friends, and the public's occasional unrealistic expectation for cure. At each of the gatherings, stories consistently underscored the importance of the work done by physicians; members were universally aligned with this belief.

Belongingness—It has been said that no man is an island. Working in a busy hospital environment can feel lonely and disconnected. The loneliness is compounded when facing a long list of tasks that must be accomplished prior to the conclusion of the day. Upon arrival at home late in the evening, the physician may find that family members are not available for an emotional connection. Belonging to a "physician family" at work, where members can speak freely and be understood, fosters a sense of connectedness and community.

Transcendence—This is one of the most powerful aspects of Finding Meaning in Medicine and is fully aligned with the Mission of AdventHealth, which is to extend Christ's healing ministry. Belief that the work is not merely one's own but that of a higher power is the strongest motivator for happiness in what one does on a daily basis, as one is acting as an intermediary for a higher power rather than as an individual. This theme, whatever the member's spiritual belief, was reliably and powerfully present in our conversations.

Cultural and Interpersonal Sensemaking—The constant influx of recurring sick patients within our acute care hospitals can lead to questions regarding the value of our work. The stories told by other physicians offered universal acclaim for the worth of what we do as healers. Often conversations revolved specifically around heartfelt descriptions of making a difference. Frequently, these were not about cures but about healing and connecting with patients, families, or hospital staff. There was a true sense that we were indeed making a difference.

One final observation . . . the beauty of the FMM experience is that it is intentionally open-ended. Attendees are invited to tell a story about "compassion" (as an example), and each speaker draws upon their reservoir of life experience to share a moment in time that likely tells us something about what is meaningful to that person. There is no rank order of meaningfulness. Meaningfulness is unique and, in its own way, sacred to every individual.

Conclusion

The Finding Meaning in Medicine storytelling experience is an investment in the well-being of individual physicians and the building/support of a culture of physician collegiality and collaboration within the hospital. The group invites physicians to share experiences and have conversations that rarely occur naturally within a busy hospital. This simple yet so very powerful group experience is a partial antidote to the numbing challenges of the practice of medicine because it invites physicians to remember the deeper meaning that drew them to medicine in the first place.

J. Michael Yurso, MD, FACS
Vice President, Evidence-Based Practice
AdventHealth

Burt Bertram, EdD, LMHC
Mental Health Counselor

Endnotes

1. Rosso BD, Dekas KH, Wrzesniewski A. On the Meaning of Work: A Theoretical Integration and Review. *Research in Organizational Behavior.* 2010;30:91-127:p. 95.

2. Rosso BD, Dekas KH, Wrzesniewski A. On the meaning of work: A theoretical integration and review. *Research in Organizational Behavior.* 2010;30:91-127:p. 93.

3. Rosso BD, Dekas KH, Wrzesniewski A. Brown, 1996. On the meaning of work: A theoretical integration and review. *Research in Organizational Behavior.* 2010;30:91-127.

4. Rosso BD, Dekas KH, Wrzesniewski A. On the meaning of work: A theoretical integration and review. *Research in Organizational Behavior.* 2010;30:91-127:pp. 103-105.

5. Rosso BD, Dekas KH, Wrzesniewski A. On the meaning of work: A theoretical integration and review. *Research in Organizational Behavior.* 2010;30:91-127:p. 107.

6. Rosso BD, Dekas KH, Wrzesniewski A. On the meaning of work: A theoretical integration and review. *Research in Organizational Behavior.* 2010;30:91-127:pp. 108-113.

7. Rosso BD, Dekas KH, Wrzesniewski A. Shamir, 1991. On the meaning of work: A theoretical integration and review. *Research in Organizational Behavior.* 2010;30:91-127.

8. Rosso BD, Dekas KH, Wrzesniewski A. Bauneister & Vohs, 2002. On the meaning of work: A theoretical integration and review. *Research in Organizational Behavior.* 2010;30:91-127.

9. Rosso BD, Dekas KH, Wrzesniewski A. On the meaning of work: A theoretical integration and review. *Research in Organizational Behavior.* 2010;30:91-127:p. 111.

10. Rothenberger DA, Rothenberger DA. Physician Burnout and Well-Being: A Systematic Review and Framework for Action. *Diseases of the Colon and Rectum.* 2017;60(6):567-576.

11. Shanafelt T, Dyrbye L, West C. Addressing Physician Burnout: The Way Forward. *JAMA.* 2017;317(9):901-902.

12. West CP, Dyrbye LN, Erwin PJ, Shanafelt TD. Interventions to prevent and reduce physician burnout: a systematic review and meta-analysis. *The Lancet*. 2016;388(10057):2272-2281.

13. Finding Meaning Discussion Groups. Remen Institute for the Study of Health and Illness. http://www.rishiprograms.org/finding-meaning-discussion-groups/. Accessed.

14. Remen RN. Finding Meaning in Medicine: Resource Guide.https://www.baystatehealth.org/-/media/files/bhy/physician-well-being/findingmeaningmedicineguide-(1).pdf?la=en. Published 2008. Accessed.

CHAPTER 15

PHYSICIAN LEADERSHIP DEVELOPMENT: INVESTING AND IMPROVING

Craig Pirner

Sy Saliba, PhD

Strong physician involvement is a critical ingredient for the success of health system initiatives. The evolution to value-based payment and "population health" only accentuates the importance of physicians who not only demonstrate clinical competence but also leadership acumen. A survey of 495 multidisciplinary leaders in health care asked, "Who are the top three most important stakeholders in your organization's response to the evolving marketplace?" Eighty-one percent of respondents chose "physicians." There was a 22-point gap between physicians and the next most popular response: "patients."[1]

Chief clinical/medical officers at health systems, charged with aligning the clinical organization in support of system strategic priorities, increasingly realize that the scope—not to mention volume!—of today's health care strategic initiatives is too complex for a single senior clinical executive to accommodate without significant support. Senior clinical executives need a cadre of physician leaders who can help to advance initiatives by, for instance, introducing and communicating changes to frontline clinicians, developing department-/specialty-specific timelines and milestones, fielding questions and concerns from the clinical ranks, problem-solving, and serving as role models. A cadre of strong physician leaders is an essential link between senior clinical executives and the responsive medical staff that organizations crave.

Despite the need, physician leadership capacity often lags behind the need for that capability. Advisory Board interviews with chief medical and quality officers make this clear:

- ⊙ "It's what we call the 'same 10 people problem.' We get the same group of physicians for X implementation as Y committee. The problem is that we don't have that next layer of physician leaders to draw from."
- ⊙ "We are spending $2.2 million annually on medical director stipends. And for what?"
- ⊙ "Some of my department chiefs are highly resistant to instilling proven quality improvement practices in their units."
- ⊙ "Medical director efficiency at my organization is uneven, at best."

So how does an organization construct an effective physician leadership development program? It takes more than money. Too often, well-intended (and sometimes expensive!) investments in physician leadership development programs fall flat. For example, programs lack a concrete link to system priorities, attendance is poor, or few new leaders emerge. Whatever the exact structure, activities, and intensity, successful cohort-based physician leadership development programs are typically disciplined about five things: (1) selecting participants, (2) developing curriculum, (3) cultivating enthusiasm, (4) encouraging on-the-job application, and (5) program execution.

Selecting Participants

A thoughtful participant selection process is critical: bad inputs, bad outputs. In deciding how to approach participant selection, organizations are balancing the individual (What physicians should be prioritized for development?) and the collective (What do we need from our physician leadership bench?). Thus, the participant selection process should reflect this balance.

Start with the collective. Use the following suggestions to help inform your philosophy about the cohort's composition:

SELECTING A PHYSICIAN COHORT	
Focus on **emerging leaders** because the governing need is to *broaden the leadership bench* by developing new leaders.	Focus on **team leaders** (i.e., physicians with defined responsibilities [even if] not supervisory per se] to lead others) because the governing need is to create a cadre of physician leaders beneath the senior clinical executive who can engage clinicians.

SELECTING A PHYSICIAN COHORT	
Focus on **individual performers** contributing to leadership activities (e.g., committees) because the governing need is to help individuals be more effective as they personally pursue results.	Focus on **interdisciplinary participants** because the governing need is to foster collaboration between physicians and non-physicians.
Focus on **leaders from a single facility or region** because the governing need is to build relations among participants who work together frequently on day-to-day issues.	Focus on **geographically dispersed leaders** because the governing need is to facilitate networking across the organization and help break silos across sites of care.

An organization must decide how to source the potential candidates. Generally, one of three models proves successful:

1. An **application** model, in which the program is announced and interested individuals submit applications.
2. A **nomination** model, in which senior leaders nominate candidates and the committee selects participants from the nominees.
3. A **selective invitation** model, in which a committee selects participants and invites them to attend absent a nomination or application.

Regardless of the participant selection model chosen, there are a variety of ways to evaluate potential "fit" for a developmental investment. Consider using, for example, organization-specific values, competency models, etc. A good place to start are these considerations (if the selection philosophy includes multidisciplinary leaders, also apply these considerations to the nursing and administrative partners who work most closely with physicians):

⊙ *Proven interest in leading*: Which physicians demonstrate interest in process and system improvement?
⊙ *Receptivity to leadership development*: Which physicians indicate an interest in receiving greater support for their leadership growth?
⊙ *Personal trajectory of the candidate*: Which physicians already hold titled leadership positions? Which physicians are likely to serve in leadership roles in the near future?
⊙ *Importance to system growth and strategic goals*: Which physicians are most critical to clinical transformation?

Once the participants have been chosen, notify them of their selection. While participation can be strongly encouraged—and, indeed, a case should be made as to why the program is worthy of the physician's time—providing physicians an opportunity to "opt out" is recommended. This reduces the risk that cohort members feel forced to participate and provides a chance for people to reveal personal factors that may limit their ability to successfully complete the program.

Developing Curriculum

There are two fundamental questions to consider: (1) What do physician leaders need to succeed in their roles? and (2) What organizational and market context informs that need?

Given the transformative change health systems are pursuing, leaders must embrace their responsibilities not only with skill but also positivity, grit, and adaptability. Thus, as the curriculum is constructed, think about the knowledge, skills, and attitudes that enable success. For example, a physician leader responsible for reducing care variation needs the *skills* to design care standards and coach peers to adopt those standards. But that leader will be even more successful when armed with *knowledge* about why care variation reduction enhances quality outcomes and an *attitude* that embraces continuous quality improvement.

Another critical decision concerns *program focus*. Most physician leadership programs aim for a relatively broad curriculum that spans multiple topics, as a leadership course at an institution of higher education might; this may also reflect that physicians need a variety of skills to succeed in their roles. To help codify *focus*, organizations might turn to their own competency models or consider the extent to which focusing on the following areas is more or less critical:

⊙ Equipping physician leaders to support the business (topics such as problem solving, financial management, goal alignment)
⊙ Increasing collaboration (topics such as team dynamics, influence, negotiation, behavior management)
⊙ Driving improvement (topics such as data-driven decisions, innovation, safety, change management)
⊙ Building culture (topics such as vision-setting, accountability, coaching)

A hierarchical curriculum model that builds on a succeeding set of course priorities is one way to address the challenge of focus. It also illustrates an aspiration that a physician's skill, as well as willingness to be engaged in the life of a hospital, grows through a more insightful grasp of leadership issues gained from the progression of courses taken.

Each layer built on a foundation of skills

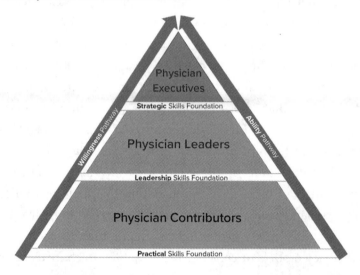

Cultivating Enthusiasm

Successfully engaging physician leaders in your leadership development program requires deliberate effort.

First, *establish a sense of prestige*. Do this by ensuring that the invitation to join the program is personalized—from a person whom physicians personally respect.

Second, *appeal to physician motivators*. Make the case for how leadership development connects to physician leaders' personal priorities. What physicians report as the biggest drivers for their engagement offers insight as to where you might begin:

⊙ Physician leaders express high desire to *influence organizational strategy.*

⊙ Physicians are motivated to *improve patient care.*

⊙ Discuss how physicians will *achieve personal growth.*

⊙ Physicians may also be motivated to *advance their career.*

Third, *secure physician commitment.* Clarify your expectations about time commitment and desired behaviors.

Fourth, *embed organizational executives.* While executive exposure is not the sole aim of leadership development programs, it often attracts physicians who desire greater insight into the personalities leading the organization and how organizational decisions are made.

Encouraging On-the-Job Application

The most effective leadership development programs extend beyond the classroom. Leaders need help as they apply the knowledge, skills, and attitudes they have learned to their day-to-day work.

This begins *in* the classroom. Articulate how the topic under consideration links to physician leader job responsibilities. Also, consider case studies and application scenarios that speak to physicians.

While it is not essential that all or even primary faculty be physicians, to the extent that physician leaders can be involved in meaningful discussions about content applicability enhances the connections made between classroom material and "real life." Encourage these physician leader contributors to reveal their successes and *struggles*. This is particularly important because physicians—accustomed to expectations of perfection—often struggle with the inherent ups-and-downs of leadership.

Execution

Saying that the program must be well-executed may seem like a blinding flash of the obvious. Yet it cannot be overstated! One would be surprised how many times the root causes of underwhelming attendance and/or declining interest is sloppy execution, such as:

- ⊙ Workshop dates being announced too close for physicians to reasonably clear their calendars.
- ⊙ Workshops being scheduled at times that ask physicians for extreme commitment. Institutions must strike a balance between preserving physician revenue generation opportunities and respecting physician human capacity.

Conclusion

The health care industry has much progress to make on physician leadership and collaboration between physician leaders and health system administrators. Given the extent to which physicians are central to care delivery, better performance is essential.

Leadership development is not a silver bullet. We must recognize that the "us versus them" sentiment that permeates the physician alignment dilemma is grounded in a true historic divide, in regulatory forces complicating attempts at shared strategy, and in misguided reduction of the dilemma to a matter of financial incentives that ignores needed investments in goodwill. We must pair physician leader development with work to clarify the scope and structure of physician leadership roles. However, leadership development can contribute significantly to reshaping health system/physician leader interactions and to filling a reservoir of goodwill. A disciplined approach to selecting participants, developing curriculum, cultivating enthusiasm, encouraging on-the-job application, and program execution will raise the likelihood of strong programmatic outcomes from institutional investment in physician leadership development.

Craig Pirner
Managing Director, Talent Development
The Advisory Board Company

Sy Saliba, PhD
Director, Leadership Institute
AdventHealth

Endnotes

1. Swensen S, Mohta NS. Leadership Survey: Physicians Come First in Achieving Change. *NEJM Catalyst*. 2017.

CHAPTER 16

A TALE OF ONE CITY: THE CINCINNATI EXPERIENCE

Herbert Schumm, MD, FAAFP

Introduction

Physician burnout exists in every community. Some systems ignore it; some combat it individually. This is a story of a community that came together to address physician burnout by promoting physician wellness.

Conception

It seemed like an innocent lunch—two doctors, a health educator, and a business professor walk into a restaurant.

After brief introductions, they realized the state of physician health was a common interest. The number of physicians affected by burnout, addiction, and suicide loomed like a gray cloud over the table. These weren't mere statistics; they were friends, neighbors, colleagues. Name after name of like-minded individuals flowed. The professor scribbled on a napkin and brought clarity to the conversation—to make a difference, we needed a continued, collaborative, expanded conversation. One physician and the educator committed to host the next meeting, an inclusive breakfast. The remaining physician picked up the tab.

This community may be like yours: hospitals ignoring or addressing a common problem individually; a medical academy trying to meet the needs of its members in a rapidly changing world while seeking to engage its professionals; physicians isolated professionally and socially, wondering why am I here? Perhaps you have a medical school and some residencies training the next generation to be well and keep up.

Convening

Breakfast it was. Spiritual care opened with a truly needed reflection and prayer. The CEO and CMO opened with their stories. Each institution told its stories and action plans. Two had well-developed medical staff wellness committees. One was driven by a letter from a fellow whose friend had died from suicide. One was working toward the Medicus Integra© Award. They each realized they all shared a passion. The conclusions were that we all had the same challenge, we needed to work together, and we were missing some key parties. We agreed to keep this going. We would invite the academy of medicine, the state physician health program, and the community mental health center.

Attendance for the second meeting doubled in size. Five health systems, a veterans' hospital, a children's hospital, the academy of medicine, physician health program, and mental health services shared more than coffee. Each brought their experiences, resources, doubts, and support. The professor needed more than a napkin but still brought clarity. We needed a purpose, a small core team to lead, and a plan for action. The purpose was to identify and create a shared strategy for addressing physician well-being that could be implemented within our community and supported by the health systems. The core team formed. The plan was yet to come.

Communication

The following meeting included brainstorming, perhaps better described as organized chaos. Two large specialty groups sent their leaders to see what was happening and support the cause. The educator and professor gracefully brought clarity again. Small groups would focus on four areas of concern:

- Physician Wellness/Counseling via Telehealth
- Primary Care Workflows Supporting Team-Based Care with Scribes/Medical Assistants
- Physician and Family Wellness Resources
- Burnout and Crisis Intervention

Each small group developed its focus area and reported back to the full group at subsequent meetings. Physician wellness and counseling by telehealth was ahead of its time and overlapped with some of the individual system employee assistance programs. The scribe/MA program explored various methods to reduce the documentation burden on physicians. While it was great to learn what each institution was implementing, synergy for the whole was missing.

While all four groups' work was important, only two were continued across the community. Physician and family resources became an opportunity for the academy to build on community events they previously sponsored. The academy led this work. They surveyed the medical community for needs and continue to provide family support.

Collaboration

Burnout and crisis intervention across all physicians presented a great need and great opportunity. The Lindner Center of

Hope is a nonprofit, full-service mental health center—a trusted community treasure. The Lindner president and one of the coalition members had a passion to build something bigger and better. The need extended beyond existing services. The health systems would support it. In honor of our veterans, the other systems would cover the VA portion of the service.

Lindner proposed a 24/7 service for rapid access plus comprehensive evaluation and treatment for any physician, medical student, resident, or fellow who called its dedicated line. Peers could recommend the service to colleagues. Wellness committees could refer physicians with confidence. The Lindner service complemented all existing resources.

The team reported utilization and common diagnoses to the large group. This enhanced the understanding of behavioral health and encouraged promotion of the service.

The team also identified an opportunity to raise awareness of physician suicide. Over 400 physicians, or one every day, die from suicide. This was more than a number, as members recounted colleagues or friends they had lost. The team partnered with the producer of *Do No Harm*, a documentary about medical student, resident, and physician suicide. The group secured rights to share the film within all member institutions. The academy sponsored the community premier for physicians and guests. This event closed with a panel consisting of the film producer, the Lindner president, and the Ohio Physicians Health Program wellness director and medical director. The robust discussion was held to a sold-out audience. The film was then available for all member institutions. Additional events were planned but postponed due to the pandemic. Nonetheless, a dialogue was opened across generations and across the community.

Connection

The group included physicians, educators, spiritual care leads, business experts, and administrators. This diversity of experience became a strength. Learning from that diversity became a connection.

The various organizations approached clinician wellness differently. We challenged each other as we learned and shared across those organizations.

Each meeting included a learning opportunity. An individual member could present information from a meeting or his own work. Outside organizations presented the work or services they offered. For example, the academy conducted a community survey and shared the results. The physician health program provided program updates and advocacy opportunities.

Other community resources shared their work. The Johnson & Johnson Human Performance Institute® presented their work to improve resilience and reduce the impact of burnout. One institution provided this service for their physician leaders. The VIA Institute on Character presented their work around the world to help people identify and live from their strengths. Several members took advantage of their free assessment.

Community

Then came a pandemic. Burnout did not decline; substance use did not plummet; and suicide risk increased. In-person meetings stopped, and the focus shifted. The group now meets virtually until it is again prudent for in-person meetings. The Lindner services are treasured even more. The learning and idea sharing are valued even more.

As the group looks to the future, they will build on their success and learning. Members consult with each other. They are expanding on pandemic challenges and learning. They are looking at institutional zero tolerance policies for substance use disorders. They are evaluating additional services for the community, organizational structure, and funding opportunities. The common need, continuous learning, and mutual support keep them together. They search for grant opportunities.

Conclusion

This is the tale of one city, so far. Your community is unique but probably has similarities.

Start today, where you are. Four people had a lunch, but their experience and passion for physician wellness started long before the lunch. They were connectors, and soon four turned into fifty. Despite no budget, the group funded mental health resources and opened a community-wide discussion on physician suicide. Are you one of the few for your community? How can you host the lunch that starts a discussion that brings your community together?

Inclusion is essential. What started as an unlikely group led to something larger than any individual. Invite and include a variety of people. Each brings an experience, a passion, and a contribution. Each person represents a unique trust and influence to support the group. It was gratifying (and surprising) to learn how many non-physicians truly cared and understood the importance of this work. The professor, educator, spiritual care lead, and academy director gave of their hearts. The non-physicians are real heroes who tread where others fear.

Learning is a glue. We may get bored with tedium and process, but we are driven to learn. Learning from each other and sharing our learning from external sources served as a cohesive bond. Plan for a learning activity at every meeting or event.

A successful meeting is organic but organized. Planning and preparation facilitate good discussion and learning. A focus on forming a complete organization may douse the flames of interest and enthusiasm. A coalition cannot and should not compete with its parent organization. Leadership must manage the balance and direct the course. Leaders assure that the work challenges when needed but always complements. The Cincinnati Coalition is not currently a legal entity but is exploring options for more formal structure. Learning, sharing, and even assuring access to critical behavioral health resources are achievable goals. More structure and formal governance are essential to conduct formal research or obtain grants.

Competitors can collaborate. Competitors often have much in common; physician well-being is one example. A few individuals brought competitors together to share resources, ideas, and energy around one challenge.

Thanks

This story involves quite a cast. A few characters must be acknowledged:

- ⊙ The professor—Daniel Geeding, PhD
- ⊙ The educator—Jan Donley, PhD
- ⊙ The first doctor—Anne Like, MD
- ⊙ The spiritual advisor—Doug Mitchell, DMin
- ⊙ The leads for mental health—Paul Samuels, MD, and Charles Bernstein, MD
- ⊙ The Lindner lead—Paul Keck, MD
- ⊙ The academy lead—Natalie Peterson
- ⊙ The physician health program—David Goldberg, MD, Craig Pratt, MD, Colleen Opremcak, MD, Nelson Heise, MA, MS

Acknowledgments

This coalition consists of several organizations. Their contributions are essential.

- ⊙ Academy of Medicine of Cincinnati (www.academyofmedicine.org)
- ⊙ Bon Secours Mercy Health (www.bsmhealth.org)
- ⊙ The Christ Hospital Health Network (www.thechristhospital.com)
- ⊙ Cincinnati Children's Hospital Medical Center (www.cincinnatichildrens.org)
- ⊙ Lindner Center of Hope (www.lindnercenterofhope.org)
- ⊙ Ohio Physicians Health Program (www.ophp.org)
- ⊙ St. Elizabeth Healthcare (www.stelizabeth.com)
- ⊙ TriHealth (www.trihealth.com)
- ⊙ UC Health (www.uchealth.com)
- ⊙ U.S. Department of Veterans Affairs (www.va.gov)

Herbert Schumm, MD, FAAFP
Vice President, Medical Director Education and Physician Engagement
Bon Secours Mercy Health

CHAPTER 17

CREATING A SAFE SPACE: THE REBIRTH OF THE PHYSICIAN LOUNGE

Ted Hamilton, MD, MBA

Introduction

Modern medical care is characterized by increasing specialization and separation of clinical services leading to physician isolation, loneliness, and burnout. Opportunities for physician communication, collaboration, and community have declined. The physician lounge, traditionally a place for physicians to gather, relax, relate, and recharge, has lost a place of prominence in many institutions. This paper calls for a revival of the physician lounge as a "safe space," intended and designed to restore the opportunity for professional connection and collegiality.

Medical Fragmentation and Physician Isolation

My eyes are not so good. I've had severe myopia (nearsightedness) since childhood. Today, I'm a grandparent with astigmatism, glaucoma, cataracts, and retinal issues causing visual floaters. Fortunately, I have good doctors who monitor my vision and under whose care I retain the ability to read and drive an automobile and watch my grandkids play sports. My glaucoma doctor referred me to one of his partners (whom he rarely sees) for cataract surgery and to a retina specialist across town for the floaters. I've benefited from outstanding care. But this is not about me. It's about my doctors and the evolution of the practice of medicine that has fragmented medical practice and separated doctors from each other.

Increasingly complex diagnostic and therapeutic capabilities have contributed to the growing specialization, sub-, and super-specialization that characterize modern medical care. Many medical specialties, such as dermatology, ophthalmology, cosmetic surgery, and even primary care disciplines, including family medicine, internal medicine, and general pediatrics, no longer require hospital-level resources to care for their patients. Doctors may go for days or weeks at a time without the opportunity to meet a colleague, to exchange pleasantries, to commiserate over mutual concerns, to relax and catch up on the kids and family.

For hospital-based physicians, such as hospitalists, intensivists, emergency physicians, surgeons, and anesthesiologists, the phenomenon of shiftwork and the demands of efficiency and productivity make it difficult to justify even a few minutes of downtime. How can I afford to take 15 or 20 minutes to relax, recoup, and re-engage with colleagues when I have five urgent consults and two new admissions waiting in the ED? How can I justify a brief, relaxed visit with a colleague when sick patients need me?

Specialization, fragmentation, and corporatization of medicine have conspired to limit physician-to-physician contact and face-to-face professional and social communication. Physicians increasingly work independently and are progressively isolated from one another. A survey of almost 1,400 practicing physicians conducted by athenahealth® in

2018 revealed that a quarter of respondents reported feeling isolated at least once a week. The study also reported a clear correlation between isolation and professional burnout.[1] Jason Horay concurs, "Physician burnout is bred in isolation and silence."[2] Another points out that "Isolation often grows during the transition from medical school, rotations, and residency to becoming a physician."[3]

Isolation often leads to loneliness. What former Surgeon General Vivek Murthy once referred to as an epidemic of loneliness in the United States has been exacerbated by the COVID-19 pandemic, with its restrictions on social interaction, masking, personal distancing, and travel. Physicians are not immune from the experience of loneliness. According to a survey reported in the *Harvard Business Review*, doctors and lawyers reported the greatest incidence of isolation and loneliness among American workers.[4] Philip Masters, MD, notes the prevalence of loneliness among physicians, remarking on the "extent to which [physicians] feel both isolated and lonely regardless of location or their professional circumstances." He also notes an association between loneliness and physician burnout.[5] Ameya Kulkarni, MD, concurs, "So the transition away from routine interaction with patients and colleagues and toward more isolated and individual activities has contributed to loneliness and resulting burnout."[6]

Time, or lack of it, appears to be a contributing factor to isolation and loneliness. It is not so much time spent in clinical activities that appears to be the major culprit, rather more the additional time required for documentation and other tasks driven by regulation and administrative duties. Richard Wenzel, MD, writing for the *New England Journal of Medicine*, opines, "Continuing to operate under the assumptions inherent in our current business model has brought us to a crisis in job satisfaction; RVU medicine and technology have conspired to cause a kind of professional loneliness." His article concludes, "I think we need uninterrupted time to reflect, to converse, and to grapple with the downsides of the unrestrained embrace of technology. Such steps could be the beginning of a journey to reclaim our profession and recapture our most treasured relationships."[7]

Loneliness has been shown to contribute to lower job satisfaction, fewer promotions, more frequent job switching, and a higher likelihood of quitting jobs.[4] There is a growing body of evidence demonstrating an association between loneliness and health status. A recent article in the *Kansas Journal of Medicine* referenced AARP® research linking loneliness to a variety of health risks, such as "high blood pressure, heart disease, obesity, a weakened immune system, anxiety, and depression."[8] Physicians do not get a pass, there is no "Get Out of Jail Free" card. Because physicians are human beings, they are subject to the same emotions and associated physical and mental manifestations of illness common to all. John J. Frey, MD, suggests that loneliness puts both doctors and patients at risk: "Professional loneliness . . . threatens the quality of clinical care by replacing personal discussions about patients but also poses risks to physician personal and professional well-being."[9]

Collegiality

In his article, "The Loneliness of Being a Physician," Gregory Hood asks, "When a physician doesn't happen across their partner, or is too overburdened with scheduling and documentation requirements to go to the hospital or attend a professional or social gathering, then what is the route of professional connectivity?"

He goes on to suggest that, "The remedy . . . is, rather simply, to congregate, to bond, to not be alone, to not be lonely."[10]

Collegiality is defined by Webster as "the sharing of authority among colleagues."[11] Medical literature reveals nuances of this definition, such as "the responsibilities of physicians to one another and to their profession"[12]; "the manner in which physicians relate to others so as to ensure that patients will be cared for properly"[12]; and "the method by which members of the collegium—the faculty and its staff—interact with each other and with the executive officer to achieve the professional goals."[13] Responsibility, relationship, interaction, and sharing are all words that evoke togetherness, fellowship, and professional interdependence. Jane Petro, MD, writes, "Collective is the operative concept in the search for collegiality."[14]

We believe that professional collegiality is a powerful antidote to physician isolation, loneliness, and professional burnout. "Collaborative teamwork involving physicians and other practice staff has been reported as a source of professional satisfaction." Also, "frequent meetings with other physicians and allied health professionals (such as business meetings . . .) fostered greater collegiality."[15] Goldstein agrees, "Regular meetings of appropriate staff at each level and between levels are absolutely essential for the sharing of information, presentation of issues, discussion of common problems, making recommendations . . . it supports the maintenance of collegiality."[13]

For generations, the physician's lounge has served as a safe place for physicians to gather, relax (if only briefly), exchange stories, obtain informal consults, laugh together, talk politics, complain (about whatever), enjoy a cup of coffee, and leave recharged. The physician lounge has provided opportunities to build relationships with other doctors and with hospital executives, a place for young doctors to become acquainted with older colleagues, a place that lends itself to meaningful interaction and encourages collaboration and collegiality.

But things are changing. An article from 2013 published in *The Atlantic*, entitled, "What Happened to the Doctors' Lounge?" opens with a brief reflection on a once-busy physicians' lounge that no longer exists, eliminated in a recent renovation.[16] An article with a similar theme by John J. Frey, MD, entitled, "Professional Loneliness and the Loss of the Doctor's Dining Room," reminisces about physician lounges as "safe places to ask questions, set plans, and learn what was important about the hospital organization, the nature of hospital management, and the long history of the place." Dr. Frey goes on to lament, "Not valuing time with other physicians or allowing for informal conversations leads to a soulless efficiency and professional isolation that drains physicians of our ability to help ourselves, help each other, and help patients." Finally, Dr. Frey calls for the creation of "safe places and time for conversation and connections."[9]

Whatever Happened to the Physician Lounge?

In many hospitals, the physician lounge has lost some of its allure. What was once a convenient respite, a place to relax with a cup of coffee and snack, to put one's feet up and catch a quick nap, has, in too many instances, become a more business-oriented facility, furnished with desks, business chairs, and computers to catch up on medical records, even bulletin boards that display comparative physician performance on quality, safety, and patient experience. Metrics are important and have their rightful place, but displaying competitive, and potentially embarrassing, data mitigates against comfort, congeniality, and community among physicians.

In other hospitals, the physician lounge has disappeared altogether. The reasons are many—inconvenient location, declining use due to physician busyness and, conversely, physicians deserting the hospital entirely to practice solely in the outpatient setting, lack of personal and social amenities, lack of attention from administration, facility renovation resulting in demolition of the lounge.

Some hospitals have chosen to open the physician lounge to a broader clientele of clinicians, such as advanced practice clinicians (APCs), nurses, and clinical administrators. There is a certain logic in affording opportunity for physicians and APCs to cross paths in a less formal, less clinical setting. After all, despite different levels of education and training, both do clinical work and carry direct patient responsibility within their training and scope. Both care for patients at the bedside, both take call, both do procedures, both document in the medical record, both write orders for patient care. But there appear to be advantages and disadvantages to this approach. On the one hand, it may contribute to cross-disciplinary team building as clinicians at various levels and across disciplines become better acquainted with each other and form relationships that contribute to mutual trust and collaboration. On the other hand, and at the risk of evoking elitism, it may compromise the potential for building camaraderie and collegiality among professional peers.

Reviving the Physician Lounge

There are many potential strategies for addressing physician isolation, loneliness, burnout, job dissatisfaction, and physician turnover—strategies that offer opportunity for physicians to experience face-to-face contact, enjoy casual conversation, make new acquaintances, interact with old friends, build connections, and enhance morale. These initiatives include relationship building during onboarding, physician mentoring, intentional peer support training, collegial reflection events (such as Rachel Remen's Finding Meaning in Medicine®), and informal social gatherings. A number of these initiatives are addressed at greater length in this book.

The physician lounge offers a "safe space" opportunity for regular, ongoing fellowship and social interaction among doctors at their own convenience and in a casual, unforced setting. Fortunately, the physician lounge, following a period of disinterest and decline, appears to be making a comeback. Health care organizations are beginning to appreciate anew the wide-ranging benefit of an attractive, comfortable, inviting "safe space" for doctors. Based on the results of a survey of staff physicians, Diane Sliwka, MD, led an effort to create a space at the University of California San Francisco (UCSF) for physicians to work and/or socialize. Dr. Sliwka says, "It's been one of the most popular interventions we've made to improve the physician work experience."[17, 18]

The following case study describes the experience of a midsized community hospital in renovating and expanding their small, outdated physician lounge and the impact that this initiative has had on physician satisfaction and culture.

Case Study: AdventHealth Sebring

AdventHealth Sebring is a 170-bed hospital serving a seasonal community of 60,000–100,000 people, located about 30 miles southwest of Orlando, Florida. The current facility opened in 1998 and included a small physician lounge added to the architectural plan almost as an afterthought. Furnishings consisted of two small desks, two chairs, and a dictating station. At most, the approximately 200 square foot space could only accommodate a maximum of two to three people at any given time and was totally inadequate for any group activity.

In 2018, plans were developed, in collaboration with the medical staff, to expand the existing space along with enhanced furnishings and services. Randy Surber, CEO, stated that the intent was to create a "home away from home" as an expression of esteem for physicians and appreciation for their commitment to patient care and loyalty to the institution. He went on to describe the engagement of physicians in the project as "palpable." Physicians were directly involved in the planning process, reviewing drawings, helping to choose furnishings and amenities. One physician noted that this project "means that you value us."

The new and improved physician lounge, which opened in late 2019, features a window wall looking out over a green lawn, studded with tall palms and bordering an azure blue lake. Amenities in the expanded space include a conference room, dictation facilities, a secluded nap room, a TV area with comfortable seating, and a kitchen with tables accommodating 36 patrons at a time. Convenient adjacencies include the medical staff administrative office, the hospitalist office, and physician parking. Refreshments are available 24 hours a day, seven days a week. Once a week, the hospital chef prepares a special noon meal for physicians, hosted by hospital administration, featuring a different cultural cuisine each week unique to the varied backgrounds of members of the medical staff.

Dr Bindu Raju, an internist/hospitalist and chief medical officer, states that most any time of the day, a stroll through the new lounge will encounter groups of three or four doctors talking, laughing, conferring, and enjoying each other's company. It is not unusual for physicians to begin and end their day's duties with a stop in the physician lounge. The "connections and bonding" between and among physicians and between administration and physicians, Surber and Raju agree, have never been stronger. While it may be difficult to measure in hard financial terms, this investment has been worth every penny.

Conclusions

The practice of medicine in the third decade of the twenty-first century has, for many physicians, become an isolated and lonely experience. Collegial connections are essential to professional satisfaction, personal well-being, and quality patient care. The well-designed and appointed physician lounge becomes a "safe space" for physician communication and relationship-building. Physician and executive leaders are encouraged to explore and take advantage of the opportunity to revive the physician lounge in the interest of physician collegiality and professional culture in the organization.

Acknowledgments

Thank you to Randy Surber, CEO of AdventHealth Sebring, and Dr. Raju Bindu, CMO, for sharing their experience of expanding and renovating the physician lounge at their hospital in Central Florida.

Ted Hamilton, MD, MBA
Chief Mission Integration Officer and Senior Vice President
AdventHealth

Endnotes

1. Hayhurst C. Disconnected: Isolation and Physician Burnout. https://www.athenahealth.com/knowledge-hub/practice-management/disconnected-isolation-and-physician-burnout. Published 2019. Accessed.

2. Horay J. How a Culture of Isolation Breeds Physician Burnout. https://curi.com/news/how-a-culture-of-isolation-breeds-physician-burnout/. Published 2019. Accessed.

3. B. S. Physician Isolation: Creating Community, Ending Stigma. In. *amopportunities.org*2019.

4. Vogel L. Medicine is one of the loneliest professions. *CMAJ: Canadian Medical Association Journal=Journal de l'Association medicale canadienne.* 2018;190(31):E946.

5. Masters MD P. The Isolation and Loneliness that Physicians Experience. https://www.kevinmd.com/blog/2019/05/the-isolation-and-loneliness-that-physicians-experience.html. Published 2019. Accessed.

6. Kulkarni A. Navigating Loneliness in the Era of Virtual Care. *The New England Journal of Medicine.* 2019;380(4):307-309.

7. Wenzel R. RVU Medicine, Technology, and Physician Loneliness. *The New England Journal of Medicine.* 2019;380(4):305-307.

8. Ofei-Dodoo S, Ebberwein C, Kellerman R. Assessing Loneliness and Other Types of Emotional Distress among Practicing Physicians. *Kansas Journal of Medicine.* 2020;13:1-5.

9. Frey J. Professional Loneliness and the Loss of the Doctors' Dining Room. *Annals of Family Medicine.* 2018;16(5):461-463.

10. Hood MD G. The Loneliness of Being a Physician. 2019. https://www.medscape.com/viewarticle/906953. Published 02/12/2019.

11. *Webster's New World Dictionary.* Second College Edition ed: Simon and Schuster; 1982.

12. Ophthalmology TECotAAo. *Collegiality. The Ethics Committee of the American Academy of Otolaryngology-Head and Neck Surgery.* Vol 115. San Francisco, California: American Academy of Ophthalmology; 1993.

13. Goldstein M. Maintenance of collegiality. *Bulletin of the New York Academy of Medicine.* 1992;68(2):308-313.

14. Petro J. Collegiality in history. *Bulletin of the New York Academy of Medicine.* 1992;68(2):286-291.

15. Friedberg MW, Peggy G. Chen, Kristin R. Van Busum, Frances M. Aunon, Chau Pham, John P. Caloyeras, Soeren Mattke, Emma Pitchforth, Denise D. Quigley, Robert H. Brook, F. Jay Crosson, and Michael Tutty. Collegiality, Fairness, and Respect. In: *Factors Affecting Physician Professional Satisfaction and Their Implications for Patient Care, Health Systems, and Health Policy.* RAND Corporation; 2013:65-72.

16. Gunderman R. What Happened to the Doctors' Lounge? *The Atlantic.* 2013. https://www.theatlantic.com/health/archive/2013/11/what-happened-to-the-doctors-lounge/281112/.

17. Zimmerschied C. Once Endangered, Doctors' Lounge Revived to Battle Burnout. https://www.ama-assn.org/practice-management/physician-health/once-endangered-doctors-lounge-revived-battle-burnout. Published 2017. Accessed.

18. Brown S. Bringing back the doctors' lounge to help fight burnout. *CMAJ : Canadian Medical Association Journal = Journal de l'Association medicale canadienne.* 2019;191(9):E268-E269.

PART III

RESTORING HOPE

HEALING THE HEART AND SOUL

I try to take care of myself. I am careful about eating right and I exercise four days a week. I'm pretty good about getting adequate sleep except for on-call interruptions. My family is important to me, but I know that clinical demands often take priority. And it never seems to be enough. I'll admit, I've never been a particularly religious person, but I've begun to wonder if there's not something missing in my life. I seem to have an itch that is difficult to scratch. And somehow, I think my story is neither unique nor isolated. When body and mind are working well, but things still don't add up, it may be time to check on the human spirit and consider time-tested methods of replenishing the need of the soul.

CHAPTER 18

"WHAT'S IN YOUR HANDS?" A PUZZLE. A THOUGHT. A PEN.
THE GIFTS OF REFLECTION AND JOURNALING

Orlando Jay Perez, MDiv

"Abu, what's in your hands?" My three-year-old granddaughter calls me "Abu."

"This is a box with a puzzle inside," I explained. Her smile filled my heart. Then I said, "Now we need to open the box, take out all the pieces, and put them together. Once we put them together, we will see this picture," pointing to the picture on the outside of the box.

Life is like a box with a puzzle inside. In order to put together the puzzle, I need to open the box and take out all the pieces. Once I place the pieces of my heart in the open, I can then start to put them together. When that happens, I can confirm if the picture on the outside of the box is the same as the pieces on the inside.

As I put together my inner stories, I have a chance to see a better picture of who I really am. This is what I refer to in this chapter as the process of reflection or journaling. Put in simple terms, "think about it, write it down."

Building puzzles requires patience and intentionality. It requires grace, because I may try to fit one piece with another piece over and over and still not find where it belongs. Puzzles require discernment and commitment because, at first, all the pieces are scattered, upside down, and disorganized. They have a diversity of shapes, colors, and connective forms and require a keen and reflective eye.

Every life is unique, just as every puzzle is unique. Every method of putting together the puzzle is also unique. Most people start with turning over all the pieces to the side where they can see parts of the picture. Some start with finding the pieces that form the frame first and begin forming the puzzle from the outside. Others look for common colors and set them in groups. There is not a right or wrong way of putting together a puzzle, but the pieces must be out of the box.

The picture on the box can be validated only when the pieces on the inside come together as one. The whole picture is then seen and appreciated. I may claim that the pieces of the puzzle form a picture of a flower, a beautiful landscape, an animal, or a famous painting. The only way to know is to risk taking the pieces out of the box and placing them together as one.

"We have *this treasure in* earthen vessels" (2 Corinthians 4:7, King James Version). The earthen vessel, the body (the box), is what holds and carries the treasure, the story, "the being" part of self. The purpose of the box is to hold the pieces of the puzzle. The purpose of the body is to hold the pieces of the heart. When the pieces come together as one, the picture of the treasure comes alive.

The treasure is the story I have been writing since the moment I was born, pieces that have formed me through the years and are stored inside the box of my heart. Reflection is the process through which the treasure within, the story that makes me who

I am, comes together within the earthen vessel and helps me see the whole person.

Health care is a discipline trained to take care of the body (the box). But the actual treasure is "inside." As important as the box is, the joy of building a puzzle is to let out the pieces and connect them as one. If I guard the box too much, for fear of letting out the pieces, I may live life without the mystery and curiosity of how a puzzle comes together.

"Think about it, write it down" is an invitation to trust my story, to connect with my inner emotions, to reflect on them, and to journal in a way that the inner treasure becomes a reflective place that can teach me, guide me, and enlighten the way I live my life. Reflecting and journaling can be the place where I take time to harmonize who I am, the story that fills my present experience and what informs it. Reflection and journaling can be places where I check to see if the puzzle has a missing piece. Thus, "We have *this treasure in* earthen vessels."

"As a man thinks *in his heart*, so is he" (Proverbs 23:7, New King James Version). An inclusive way of reframing this text is, "As humans think **in their hearts**, so are they." Again, here is a reference to the importance of paying attention to what is inside the heart. French philosopher René Descartes wrote in 1637, "I think, therefore, I am."[1] Descartes forgot that between the "I think" and the "I am" is "the heart."

The notion that "thinking" happens in "the heart" brings an important principle of reflection: emotions and feelings precede what I think. Why is this important? Because human emotions and vulnerability reside in the heart. Our emotions translate into thoughts, and thoughts translate into words/language. Language translates into communication venues such as body language, verbal language, and written language.

When babies are born, they bring the capacity to feel before they can think, speak, and develop language. As we mature, we lose vulnerability and use rationality to protect the inner emotions that make us human.

According to the creation story, God formed the first earthen vessels in God's own image. The material for the earthen vessels was "dust of the ground." Then God put his own breath into that earthen vessel, and it became the treasure, "a living being" (Genesis 2:7, New King James Version).

Sadly, the open vulnerability and transparency Adam and Eve enjoyed with each other became compromised. Shame, blame, and guilt drove them away from their authentic selves. The wholeness of life and vulnerability, intended for humans to be the place where the fullness of love and relationships live, became compromised by the need to hide and guard their inner hearts.

Taking out the pieces of their inner puzzle, their hurting hearts, became scary. Their idea of "being safe" was to cover up self rather than open their hearts. Shame drove them away from each other and from who they were.

The healing process began through an invitation to reflect, a kind of journaling experience. The first reflective encounter recorded in scripture is found in Genesis 3:9–11, and it began with a three-word question: "Where are you?" The reflective conversation was followed by a second question, "Who told you?" It was as if God was saying, "Let's open the box and see the pieces." God invited the first couple to a place of vulnerability and transparency. In order to see the picture, all the pieces needed to be out in the open. "Think about it, write it down."

Reflection is a process based more on questions than answers. It is an open process, concerned with curiosities rather than solutions. It sustains the need to figure out life and invites the inner heart to be surprised with the simple ways of being human.

In his book, *The Reflective Practitioner*, Donald A. Schön writes, "Many practitioners, locked into a view of themselves as technical experts, find nothing in the world of practice to occasion reflection. They become too skillful at techniques of selective inattention, junk categories, and situational control, techniques which they use to preserve the constancy of their knowledge-in-practice. For them, uncertainty is a threat; its admission is a sign of weakness."[2]

What are some of the benefits that come from reflecting and journaling?

Soulfulness

When I sit down to write, I invite myself to slow down, turn off the inner noise in my head, and hear the quiet insights of my heart. The word "insight" means "to see in." When I see in, intimacy (in-to-me see) with self becomes a possibility. Intimacy is a close encounter with our "soul or spirit."

I love the way Thomas Moore puts it: "'Soul' is not a thing, but a quality or a dimension of experiencing life and ourselves. It has to do with depth, value, relatedness, heart, and personal substance. Care of the Soul begins with observance of how the soul manifests itself and how it operates. *We can't care for the soul unless we are familiar with its ways.*"[3]

Becoming familiar with my inner heart touches the multiple pieces of the human puzzle and helps me see who I am as a person. Through reflection, observation, and journaling, I connect with the texture, colors, shapes, and sizes of the stories that form my picture.

Self-awareness

Who I am informs what I do, whether or not I like it. The process of "becoming aware" of who I am does not happen in the "doing" or "knowing" domain but in the "being" domain. Thus, I am called a "human being," not "a human doer" or "a human knower."

I may not know who I am. But writing down what I think provides a mirror to see a reflection of myself. The development of self-awareness then gives me a chance to invite change and future into my present experience.

"Each of us has an inner teacher that is an arbiter of truth, and each of us needs the give-and-take of community in order to hear that inner teacher."[4] When I find a community with which I can trust to share my inner self, the process of self-awareness is enhanced and blessed. The fresh eyes of other people can sometimes help me see blind spots or pieces of my inner puzzle that I may not see on my own. Besides, it can be fun to build puzzles or self-reflect with those I trust and with whom I have relationships.

Empathy

In 1924, psychiatrist Harry Stack Sullivan developed a concept for psychiatric interventions based on one core principle: "Everyone is much more simply human than otherwise."[5] My capacity to have empathy for other human beings is proportional to the capacity to have empathy for myself. Reflection and journaling give me a safe place to let my human emotions and experiences be written and seen through personal eyes, which can then extend compassion and grace to what gets revealed.

When human empathy comes from within, I have authority and personal power to let go of external pressures that create unhealthy models of self-esteem. Parker Palmer brings it home when he writes, "Power works from the outside in, but authority works from the inside out."[4]

Wisdom

There is a basic difference between wisdom and intelligence. Intelligence, knowledge, and information are valued traits essential for some critical areas of life. Wisdom is more about pausing and reflecting on the values that make life meaningful. The practice of reflection invites me to appreciate the simple moments of my life and differentiate between those things that seem urgent and those that are important.

"The extent of our capacity for reciprocal reflection in action [think of it, write it down] can be discovered only through an action science which seeks to make what some of us do on rare occasions into a dominant pattern of practice."[2]

Wholeness

The journey of wholeness is an invitation to live a life of harmony that integrates body, mind, and spirit as one. When it comes to attention to the spirit, reflection on key spiritual indicators such as love, joy, and peace can provide a canvas on which I can assess relationships, meaning and purpose, and the stillness of a peaceful spirit.

Reflective questions such as, "Who are the people who love me and care for me?"; "What brings joy to my life?"; and "What gives me a sense of peace today?" provide a personal mirror where I can explore the balance of a meaningful and fulfilled life.

Transformation

Reflection elevates the human being from "formation" (who I am) and "information" (who I say I am) into "transformation" (who I can become). This is where the fear and hope of inner vulnerability within a reflective process can bring grace and change to my life.

I close with the words of Thomas Moore, who summarizes what I have shared in a beautiful statement: "Living artfully might require something as simple as *pausing*. Some people are incapable of being arrested by things because they are always on the move. A common symptom of modern life is that there is no time for thought or even for letting impressions of a day sink in. Yet it is only when the world enters the heart that it can be made into soul. The vessel in which soul-making takes place is an inner container scooped out by reflection and wonder. There is no doubt that some people could spare themselves the expense and trouble of psychotherapy simply by giving themselves a few minutes each day for quiet reflection."[3]

"Abu, what's in your hands?" A simple question from a three-year-old little girl filled with curiosity and wonder.

"This is a box with a puzzle inside. Now we need to open the box, take out all the pieces, and put them together. Once we put them together, we will see this picture."

Are you ready to see your picture? Think of it, write it down!

Orlando Jay Perez, MDiv
Vice President, Mission & Ministry
AdventHealth

Endnotes

1. Dictionary.com. The New Dictionary of Cultural Literacy. In: Houghton Mifflin Harcourt Publishing Company; 2005.

2. Schön DA. *The Reflective Practitioner: How Professionals Think in Action*. USA: Basic Books, Inc.; 1983.

3. Moore T. *Care of the Soul: An Inspirational Programme to Add Depth and Meaning to Your Everyday Life*. New York, USA: HarperCollins Publishers; 1992.

4. Palmer PJ. *The Courage to Teach: Exploring the Inner Landscape of a Teacher's Life*. San Francisco, CA, USA: Jossey-Bass; 1998.

5. Sullivan HS. *Concepts of Modern Psychiatry*. New York, USA: W. W. Norton & Company, Inc.; 1953.

CHAPTER 19

PRAYER. MINDFULNESS. MEDITATION. PEACE.

Malcolm Herring, MD
Rachel Forbes Kaufman

Introduction

A step toward peace is a step toward healing. The healing professions have not experienced much peace lately. The national dialogue in medicine is currently dominated by physician burnout and the COVID-19 pandemic. What we focus on, we move toward. If we focus on burnout, we will move toward burnout. If we want peace to adorn the heart of practice, we must move toward well-being. If we want to transform the heart, we must work on the heart. Prayer, mindfulness, and meditation are the most effective tools for transformation. In this chapter, we will look at these tools, more from the perspective of a practitioner than an authority, and we will highlight the powerful role of these spiritual practices in the healing art. Ironically, these practices are only minor considerations in wellness committees and well-being conferences across the United States. Whatever the reason for any neglect, these tools belong in the well-being toolkit.

What follows was written for people who provide patient care. While this is written from the perspective of a Christ follower, virtually every practice has its counterpart in the great faith traditions. I urge you to find the practices that work for you, within your familiar tradition. Of course, if we dedicated this entire book to any one of these practices, we would not cover the subject. So, take what works. Leave what does not, and be reassured that helpful resources abound.

Peace

When do we have well-being? The simplest explanation is that people, even physicians, experience well-being when they experience meaning and purpose. How do people find what gives them meaning and purpose? Sometimes an influential person in their life helps them define their role. Sometimes they are inspired by books or movies. People of faith often speak of "call." The concept of call is that the Creator confers a person's meaning and purpose. How do you discover your call or your purpose? How can you know that you are on the right track? What can derail you? Derailed purpose is not uncommon. Dejection and burnout happen when we lose sight of our purpose. Distractions, isolation, irritation, and overwork are familiar culprits, and our relationships are the casualties—relationships with our patients, physician colleagues, God, scripture, families, and government. Here are three steps toward restoring relationships.

Prayer

Prayer is an ancient practice, often resisted in postmodern thinking. Prayer comes in many forms. Some examples are supplication, intercession, adoration, thanksgiving, and meditation. Supplication is asking for God to supply something, maybe a needed medication or a cross-matched unit of packed cells. Intercession is asking God to help someone else, quite often a patient. Intercessory prayer **for** a patient can be done easily in a private moment, but prayer **with** a patient requires us to invite the patient into the prayer. Many physicians I have met[1] are reluctant to make that invitation out of fear of creating a social gaffe, but 50 percent of seriously ill patients are receptive to a prayer invitation.[2] Most of my preoperative patients were visibly relieved to have shared a prayer with their surgeon.

Inviting patients to pray must be done carefully and with sensitivity to their clinical status, faith tradition, and apparent openness. Certainly, not every patient is appropriate for such an invitation. We believe that the more we have God's Spirit working in us, the more attuned we will be to the patient's desire for invited prayer. However, once we have cleared that hurdle, there are health benefits for the patient. For instance, prayer can improve pain tolerance, especially for religious patients.[3] It has been shown to reduce stress in Muslim chemotherapy patients.[4]

Prayers of adoration express awe and praise for God's work. For instance, it is awe-inspiring to ponder wound healing and the complex cellular and chemical events that make it happen. Who could possibly design such a process? Thanksgiving may be the most important prayer form for physician well-being. Paul of Tarsus advised that we should pray and give thanks in all circumstances.[5] Prayers of gratitude slowly change our own attitudes and especially soften our default response to events. We need little coaching to utter a "Thank God!" with a sigh of relief when you get that unit of packed cells in the operating room as the patient's blood pressure drops. However, even more likely to change our attitudes are prayers expressing thanks for "little" things and routine services. Maybe more beneficial to us yet is praying thanks for "hard things," situations, and people that challenge us but help lead us toward spiritual and emotional growth. Finally, meditation is different from these other prayer forms in that it emphasizes listening or quiet rather than talking.

Mindfulness

Mindfulness includes several kinds of practices that seek to increase awareness and to reduce stress. All the practices involve giving full attention to something that is present with you in this very moment, things like breathing, walking, eating, singing, laughing, etc. Suppose we took a mindful walk. We would practice an intense awareness of each slow step, noting how the grass crunches beneath our weight, how the shoe looks and feels, the aromas that fill your nose, and any emotions you might feel. If the mind wanders, bring it back to the awareness of walking. The mind and the body should be in synergy with each other. The essence of mindfulness is a focus on now, sustaining an awareness of the very moment. If you choose to focus on your breathing, choose a quiet, comfortable place with subdued lighting. A mindfulness session is often done while seated. It can be done alone or in a group. There are mindfulness guides available on the internet that add soothing music and visual images, although these are not necessary to the practice.

The benefits that people report after practicing mindfulness are that they feel peace, contentment, and wholeness. Some report that they simply feel rested. Of course, mindfulness is not limited to predetermined practice sessions. You can apply mindfulness principles all through your day. As you do, people in your sphere feel validated by your presence to them and that you have built a default attitude of appreciation.

A technique you can try is called Loving Kindness.[6] It is a way to direct love and compassion to yourself, loved ones, and even enemies.

1. Sit and calm your mind.

2. Call to mind someone you love easily without a lot of conflict in your lives. Visualize them and then yourself, saying to them, "I wish you to be well, I wish you to be happy, and I wish you to be fulfilled (or to transcend suffering or to live with ease)."

3. Bring to mind someone you do not know as well. Picture them in your mind, and picture yourself telling them the same phrases.

4, Picture in your mind someone with whom you have difficulty, and visualize yourself saying the same to them.

5. Bring yourself to mind. Look in the mirror and give yourself that same compassion.

6. Expand those same sentiments out to the whole world, to a large group of people.

7. Sit until you are ready to move on with your day.

Loving Kindness is opening our hearts for others, so that our hearts can find peacefulness.

Are there any measurable effects of mindfulness? One example is a psychometric study of senior medical students who used an audio CD of guided mindfulness practice daily for eight weeks that significantly reduced stress and anxiety based on the Perceived Stress Scale (PSS) and the Depression, Anxiety and Stress Scale (DASS). This effect was maintained for eight weeks after the intervention.[7] Moreover, structural changes in the brain have been attributed to mindfulness practice. Marchand provides a comprehensive review of structural studies. Interestingly, because of variations in methodology, the results of the studies are not uniform, but medial frontal regions of the brain were the most consistently affected, including the anterior cingulate cortex.[8] Mindfulness impacts regions of the brain that govern attention, emotional regulation, and thinking patterns.

Meditation

Meditation and mindfulness are different. Where mindfulness fills the mind with a greater awareness, building synergy between mind and body, meditation narrows awareness and calms the mind. There are different kinds of meditation, including breath awareness, visualizations, and guided meditation.[9] O H2O positron emission tomography (PET) is a tool to quantitate blood flow that reveals increased flow during meditation in the dorso lateral and orbital frontal cortex, anterior cingulate gyri, and other regions associated with the so-called executive attentional network.[10] Functional magnetic resonance imaging[11,12] and single-photon emission computerized tomography (SPECT) scanning[13] confirm the PET scan findings, and electroencephalography[14] also shows increased activity.[11] C-raclopride PET scanning detected a 69 percent increase in dopamine release in the ventral striatum, a phenomenon associated with a decreased readiness for action.[9] Much of brain physiology remains a mystery, and we can expect more from science in the future.

Meditation is at least a 5,000-year-old spiritual practice, which was adopted early within the Christian tradition to achieve union with God.[15-17] Skepticism of the spiritual practice arose during both the Spanish Inquisitions and the Protestant Reformation,[18] but most of the resurgence in the Western world in the last several decades resulted from Eastern influences in the New Age Movement of the 1960s and 1970s. More recently, however, Father Thomas Keating and others have sought to restore meditation to a form of contemplative prayer called "centering prayer."

Your authors offer basic directions to help you begin a centering prayer practice but would refer you to a much richer explanation in Keating's seminal book,[19] and to extensive literature, for guidance on other kinds of meditation. At the beginning, Keating recommends selecting a sacred word. We use the word "love" because it is a prominent feature of the Spirit of God in our tradition, and it becomes a kind of "shorthand" to use to invoke the Spirit of God during centering prayer.

There are different ways to start, all designed to focus. Some will call to mind a particular word, prayer, or saying. The length of any one session is commonly 20 to 30 minutes. If you intend to continue more than 30 minutes, plan for a break. You can use a mindfulness practice to create a five-minute break. Try walking slowly and mindfully, focusing your attention on each step. We favor meditating daily for 20 minutes or more for optimal benefits. Be patient with yourself, as we believe that benefits will not be fully appreciated until at least 30 days' practice have accrued.

There are three impediments to meditation: sleepiness, random thoughts, and blocking because of some anxiety, such as PTSD. Here are four strategies to avoid unwanted sleep. Treat yourself to eight hours of sleep each night. Take a short nap before you start your session if you feel sleepy. Avoid sessions just after you awaken in the morning or just before you go to bed at night or right after a meal. Avoid a too comfortable or reclining chair. An upright posture will help remind you if you are falling asleep.

Random thoughts are not bad. They are just a part of the way our brains work. Occasionally, the content of the thoughts can be disturbing. This is just your brain trying to throw out the garbage. Some people avoid meditations because the practice can trigger unpleasant memories or physical sensations associated with PTSD, but, with practice and the help of a meditation guide or a spiritual companion, blocking can be addressed.

As you start to meditate, pay close attention to each breath; notice the air as it passes through your nose and mouth; notice the restful, momentary pause between exhaling and inhaling. Simply directing your attention to breathing serves to block many potential random thoughts. Yet, thoughts will still get through. How you handle a thought is important. You do not want to invite the thought in for "coffee." Nor do you want to violently suppress the thought. Deal with thoughts gently, just like you want to deal with the other things in your life. Imagine your invading thought being enveloped by your sacred word. Try not to decide if the thought is bad or good. Imagine the thought going off in the distance or floating by on a boat or riding by in a car. Just acknowledge that "there is a thought" and let it go. Return your attention to your breath.

Guaranteed, one of these two thoughts will come up: "I wonder how much more time do I have? Isn't this session about over?" Set an alert for the end of the session. Then you will not have to be concerned about going over time. If you are in a group, the leader might start and end the session with a chime. Each of us uses a pleasant soft chime from the ringtone menu on our cell phones. When your session ends, open your eyes slowly. Take a few breaths, then a few steps, and return to your usual activities, taking your peace with you.

Over time, you will train your physiology to respond to events with greater peace. You will enjoy a conditioned response to your breath and to your sacred word. As you move from one activity to another during the day, take a few seconds to consciously breathe and recall your sacred word.

Peace is contagious. Your patients and staff will start to be "infected." They will begin to notice that you have a more measured reaction to events. You will have rehearsed letting go of thoughts so much that it will become second nature to you. The ancient spiritual masters regarded this as a positive spiritual discipline and referred to it as "detachment."

Some wonder if centering prayer is really prayer since so little is said. Centering prayer is the prayer of grace. It cedes all priorities, desires, and needs to God. It is the prayer of faith, relying on God to impart what he wants directly to our hearts without passing through our mental bias. It is the prayer of peace where we learn to rely on Him.

Conclusion

The practice of medicine is assailed by things like pandemics, insufficient personal protective equipment, electronic medical records, malpractice suits, racial conflicts, government caprice, and noncompliant patients. We certainly can combat each of these problems, but, invariably, more problems will come to take their place. Evidence supports that physician well-being leads to patient well-being. When we apply the tools of science, we can see that peace changes our neurons and our behaviors. Our professional experience in health care suggests that well-being happens when people experience meaning, purpose, and joy in their lives. Whatever the magnitude of problems, prayer, mindfulness, and meditation can bring our hearts, minds, and actions into alignment. And when we are fully integrated and aligned, medicine will finally be transformed into a robust healing art.

Acknowledgments

The authors gratefully acknowledge the thoughtful advice of John Hill of Zionsville, IN, Peggy Herring, and William Turnbull of Midway, UT.

Malcolm Herring, MD
Vascular Surgeon
Independent

Rachel Forbes Kaufman
Spiritual Counselor
Forbes Consulting

Endnotes

1. Sulmasy D. *The Healer's Calling: A Spirituality for Physicians and Other Health Care Professionals*. United States: Paulist Press; 1997.

2. MacLean CD, Susi B, Phifer N, et al. Patient Preference for Physician Discussion and Practice of Spirituality: Results From a Multicenter Patient Survey. *Journal of General Internal Medicine*. 2003;18(1):38-43.

3. Dezutter J, Wachholtz A, Corveleyn J. Prayer and pain: the mediating role of positive re-appraisal. *Journal of Behavioral Medicine*. 2011;34(6):542-549.

4. Rezaei M, Adib-Hajbaghery M, Seyedfatemi N, Hoseini F. Prayer in Iranian cancer patients undergoing chemotherapy. *Complementary Therapies in Clinical Practice*. 2008;14(2):90-97.

5. Tarsus Po. The First Epistle of Paul to the Thessalonians. In: *New King James Bible*. Thomas Nelson, Inc. ; 1982.

6. Keltner D. *Born to Be Good: The Science of a Meaningful Life*. New York, New York, USA: W. W. Norton Company; 2009.

7. Warnecke E, Quinn S, Ogden K, Towle N, Nelson MR. A randomised controlled trial of the effects of mindfulness practice on medical student stress levels: Effects of mindfulness practice on student stress levels. *Medical Education*. 2011;45(4):381-388.

8. Marchand W. Neural mechanisms of mindfulness and meditation: Evidence from neuroimaging studies. *World Journal of Radiology*. 2014;6(7):471-479.

9. Kjaer TW, Bertelsen C, Piccini P, Brooks D, Alving J, Lou HC. Increased dopamine tone during meditation-induced change of consciousness. *Cognitive Brain Research.* 2002;13(2):255-259.

10. Lou H, Kjaer T, Friberg L, Wildschiodtz G, Holm S, Nowak M. A 15O-H2O PET study of meditation and the resting state of normal consciousness. *Human Brain Mapping.* 1999;7(2):98-105.

11. Lazar SW, Bush G, Gollub RL, Fricchione GL, Khalsa G, Benson H. Functional brain mapping of the relaxation response and meditation. *NeuroReport.* 2000;11.

12. Ritskes R, Ritskes-Hoitinga M, Stodkilde-Jørgensen H, Baerentsen K, Hartman T. MRI Scanning during Zen Meditation; the picture of enlightenment. *Constructivism in the Human Sciences.* 2003;8:85-90.

13. Newberg A, Alavi A, Baime M, Pourdehnad M, Santanna J, d'Aquili E. The measurement of regional cerebral blood flow during the complex cognitive task of meditation: a preliminary SPECT study. *Psychiatry Research: Neuroimaging.* 2001;106(2):113-122.

14. Hirai T. *Zen Meditation and Psychotherapy.* Japan Publications Inc.; 1989.

15. Ruusbroec J. *The Spiritual Espousals and Other Works.* New Jersey, USA: Paulist Press; 1985.

16. Ponticus E. *On Prayer, One-Hundred and Fifty-Three Texts, The Philokalia.* Vol 1. London, UK: Faber and Faber; 1979.

17. Climacus J. *The Ladder of Divine Ascent.* New York, New York, USA: Paulist Press; 1982.

18. Ewer FC. *Catholicity in Its Relationship to Protestantism and Romanism.* In: G.P. Putnam's Sons; 1896.

19. Keating T. *Open Mind, Open Heart: The Contemplative Dimension of the Gospel.* New York, New York, USA: Continuum International Publishing Group; 1994.

CHAPTER 20

A JOURNEY OF CONNECTION

Kathleen Gibney, PhD, LP, ABPP

Introduction

"I define connection as the energy that exists between people when they feel seen, heard, and valued; when they can give and receive without judgment; and when they derive sustenance and strength from the relationship. Courage starts with showing up and letting ourselves be seen."   *~ Brené Brown*

Many have influenced my way of showing up in the world. My mother, maternal grandmother, and paternal aunts are the voices and stories I often share from my heart. Professionally, mentors and mentees continue to teach that my authentic self is necessary in all that I do. And two women, Rachel Naomi Remen and Brené Brown, have validated my intuition, family stories, and professional paradigm. Rachel Naomi Remen, MD, is a physician and writer whose personal struggle with Crohn's disease informed her approach to life and her study of medicine. How physicians and others understand illness and health and how body and mind are intimately involved in the art of medicine have been heavily influenced by her leadership. Brené Brown, PhD, LMSW, is a world-renowned research professor at the University of Houston Graduate College of Social Work where she has rigorously studied, published, and spoken about vulnerability, courage, authenticity, and shame. Her research findings and use of narrative have highlighted the importance of living life in the present compassionately. These voices have been transformative in my reflection of the art of practicing medicine and in the creation of a frame of reference for my journey of walking with physicians, advanced practice providers (APPs), health care administrators and, recently, health care workers across the spectrum, before and during the Coronavirus Disease 2019 Pandemic (COVID-19). And, as the world attempts to create a new normal, I am aware that all the voices of my life journey continue to offer hope that we will find ways to be present, to connect, to heal, by seeing, hearing, and valuing one another.

This chapter attempts to examine how the work of providing well-being programming, as it is presently formulated, is not enough. Current well-being programming is not enough to try to meet the needs of those who are limited by their training to identify what they need. These people often struggle to access available resources for fear of the consequences of a stigmatizing system. Furthermore, the pandemic laid bare the fact that health care delivery itself has pushed people to the limits of their abilities to stand in the current system without experiencing trauma or moral injury. A new structured and well-developed plan grounded in the reality of the deficits of health care delivery is required, as well as an acknowledgement of the real consequences of training health care professionals through shaming and creating a sense of being "different from others." And without opportunities for all employees to be valued for their contributions, regardless of what those contributions are, we will likely see unprecedented levels of mental health challenges impacting our health care system from inside the ranks of those we rely on to care for us.

Name the Reality of the Work

"The expectation that we can be immersed in suffering and loss daily and not be touched by it is as unrealistic as expecting to be able to walk through water without getting wet." ~ Rachel Naomi Remen

Before COVID-19, my role as director of the Center for Physician Well Being (CPW) for a large Central Florida health care organization, along with my small team, was to support physicians, APPs, and their families. Many needed to be seen, heard, and valued, highlighted by the fact that many described themselves as "invisible" in the mainstream medical model that is "largely defined by the transactional diagnostic and therapeutic services to patients' problems . . . rather than relation-based models of service."[1]

Through an immersion model, including hospital and outpatient settings, CPW created trusted partnerships and provided resources to teams, residency programs, and departments. We learned a great deal about how physicians are trained to believe they must be perfect, expect perfection from others, show no human needs or emotion, and to put patients and their role as doctor before all else. We learned they judged themselves harshly with language reflecting not being good enough. In addition, we became aware that an entire system of knowing oneself was not accessible to them. This lack of knowledge of a full self is the result of a "conspiracy" of influences and dynamics that begins well before medical school and is heightened at every moment of technical training and medical professional socialization. They struggled to identify body language—both their own and others—and to find words to label their emotions and thoughts. A great irony appeared to exist. As much as physicians and APPs told us how much they wanted to be seen, heard, and valued, they confided that they hid their authentic selves (and certainly their emotions) to "survive in the system." When they were able to see emotions as another source of information to interpret and use, many began to find new ways of caring for their patients and themselves.

Then, in the fall of 2019, I retired, only to be invited back when COVID-19 reached pandemic levels. I was contracted to provide psychological consultation with a diverse group of hospital employees to identify resources, to communicate coping strategies, and to create and deliver education and support services to all employees. It became apparent that this emergency was different from all others in that, regardless of the position one held in the organization, the pandemic was making itself known. There were more questions than answers, and there was no end in sight. An intensive care unit nurse manager spoke most succinctly about the needs across the organization when she voiced the sentiment, reminiscent to me from physicians and APPs in the past: "People just need to be seen and heard."

Shanafelt, Ripp, & Trockel[2] found health care professionals presented with five requests to organizations during COVID-19: hear me, protect me, prepare me, support me, and care for me. Or put another way, "to be seen, heard, and valued." In addition, the authors suggest that team members must be encouraged to ask for help when needed, to rely on each other, and to defer less important and time-sensitive activities. In this short and non-evidence-based summary of common-sense strategies, as well as the forced adaptations that the pandemic created, we may have the most succinct description of what is needed to build a foundation for a better future: create a culture of safety, learning, diversity, authentic presence, and connection. Most importantly, it must come from allowing people to be heard and seen so that one can define what that culture looks like from the view of those who would benefit from it.

Certainly, in the work our team participated in during the pandemic, we found the greatest impact of our endeavors came when two licensed mental health counselors from CPW were dispatched to the COVID-19 units. The intent was to create a presence with the teams at their morning and evening huddles where they would simply be present, give stress-management tips (e.g., breathing exercises or reframing practices), and then be available to listen. Some adjustments were able to be made in the daily lives of the staff according to the feedback the counselors shared with supervisors in a confidential manner. In addition, rounds that provided information, stress-reduction tips, and time for concerns saw steps implemented to ensure a higher sense of safety among the staff of food and environmental services. Day after day, the message from those who were involved reported that having "just those few minutes of connection was life-giving."

But here, too, a culture of shame about not being good enough emerged with people feeling they should be doing more: more for patients, more for team members, more for the community, more for their families. Some spoke of themselves as the one who needed to keep going for everyone else, as if they were machines that must keep producing. But even machines need down time for maintenance. To judge oneself as never good enough, especially when situations and circumstances are largely out of one's control, is not in service to anyone. To have a goal of being a compassionate caregiver and yet hold oneself to unattainable standards, is a practice in self-destruction. Joyce Rupp[3] speaks about compassionate care in the following way: "It can take many long years of living compassionately before we stop counting the cost and respond with fewer regrets or self-concerns. This is not to say that we omit taking care of ourselves or deny our own feelings. Far from it. It is the person who knows how to care well for self who will offer the purest and most generous compassion to another. We are, after all, to love others as we love ourselves."

The delivery of compassionate health care demands that individuals, teams, and organizations that provide that care set attainable goals, practice self-care, and create cultures that respect human dignity for themselves and the people they serve. Without those efforts, I believe health care workers will continue to feel as though they are drowning in a sea of indifference and disrespect for their efforts.

Share Our Human Experience

"The most basic and powerful way to connect to another person is to listen. Just listen. Perhaps the most important thing we ever give each other is our attention . . . A loving silence often has far more power to heal and to connect than the most well-intentioned words."

~ Rachel Naomi Remen

Not too long into the pandemic, I received a call from a physician who had reached out to me two years before to share a story that he explained was about an encounter with a friend. During the encounter, he realized that a retreat where we practiced active listening had affected the outcome of their discussion. He requested that the story and active listening tips be included in my monthly newsletter. Now, as the pandemic was impacting everyone's life, he called again to share another story. But let me start with sharing how the first story appeared in the newsletter.

The other day I received a phone call from a physician; I will call him Dr. Fix-it. He wanted to know if the two of us could meet over a cup of coffee. I am always interested in sharing a cup of coffee or tea, as it reminds me of time spent with my grandparents around our old kitchen table just listening to adult conversations. So, of course, we arranged to meet, and the conversation quickly turned to a recent visit he had with his old friend, Jack. Dr. Fix-it explained that he and Jack were reminiscing when his friend became quiet. Dr. Fix-it shared the rest of the story something like this: I immediately started to fill in the silence, talking about my family and some crazy stories from work. I was aware that I thought it was unusual for Jack to be so quiet, but I just kept talking.

After several minutes, Jack looked at me directly and said, "I have something I really want to talk about, but you aren't making it easy." Dr. Fix-it said he remembered that at that moment he looked at his friend, and said, "So just spit it out already." Dr. Fix-it reported that he noticed that Jack sighed before he began to speak slowly and quietly, sharing that he had recently received a devastating health diagnosis and that his wife of many years had said she didn't know if she could stay with him as he went through the treatment. Dr. Fix-it shared that he immediately said, "Well we can figure it out. I know some people who can help with treatment options, you know that. And my wife and I can talk to your wife; we know good lawyers if it comes to that," and on and on. He reported that Jack just sat there, still and quiet. Tears filled his friend's eyes, and Dr. Fix-it said, I just kept saying things like, "It's okay. You will figure it out and I can help." After a few more minutes, Jack said, "Okay, I guess I will just get going now and I'll call you soon." Dr. Fix-it said he felt terrible. "I felt like I was failing badly." He said then I thought about our retreat and active listening, and I realized I needed to shift from fixing to listening.

Dr. Fix-it said he reached out and touched his friend's arm and said, "Jack, let's start at the beginning, and please tell me all that you know and what it has been like for you learning about all of this." He said Jack looked at him for a second longer and then started to tell him the whole story. Dr. Fix-it said he didn't speak again for several minutes, only nodded, and grunted occasionally. After Jack had finished his story, Dr. Fix-it asked a couple of questions and listened more. He told me he once again touched his friend's arm and said, "I am so sorry that you have been living with all of this alone for this long. I am sorry I wasn't listening." He said Jack smiled and simply said, "But you are listening now, and I can't thank you enough for that, my friend!" How many times do we find ourselves in the position of Dr. Fix-it, thinking we need to help or fill a silence or void in the conversation? And how many times are we Jack where we desperately need to be heard and nothing more?

That was the story as Dr. Fix-it wanted it to be shared in the newsletter along with tips for active listening. Now during the pandemic, he shared once again that learning to stop fixing and start listening has continued to impact his life. He wanted me to know that his oldest daughter had recently spent two hours talking about how she felt trapped at home and finding it hard to be separated from her friends and do her schoolwork. He said it was all just what you would expect from a teenage girl right now. But then his daughter said to him, "Thanks, Dad, for listening to me go on and on. I know you have a hard job and you are tired, but I want you to know that I know I can tell you anything now. It is really good." Dr. Fix-it said to me, "I got teary when she said that, and she laughed and said, 'Come on, Dad, don't get all mushy on me.'" He said, "Isn't life a hoot? I guess I just wanted you to know I am still learning, and I keep practicing."

Most physicians are familiar with the saying, "learn one, do one, teach one." There are few places, however, in the entire enterprise of medicine where focused attention is given to learn, do, and teach listening and connection. This doctor reminded me that I am grateful that we created such spaces.

Create Safe Places for Diverse Dialogue

"Perhaps the secret of living well is not in having all the answers but in pursuing unanswerable questions in good company."

~ *Rachel Naomi Remen*

Why is it important for us to understand that physicians and nurses are taught to focus on finding answers and fixing problems? Primarily, the expectation that they will have such answers sets them apart from others. In the past, it put them on a pedestal that has been shaken by Google and expansive access to medical knowledge (factual and not) and challenges their status in the community. It is no longer adequate for medical experts to have medical information and access to treatment options. Now they need to know how best to connect in meaningful ways to individual patients and their families and play an active role in helping them decide and implement optimal treatment.

The Patient Experience movement was aware that patients needed a voice and wanted to be seen as people, not just diagnosed. This movement has responded to consumer and funding demands by focusing on teaching empathy-based listening skills, largely by providing scripts and short training periods for providers at every level. Overall, patients have noted an improvement in being a part of their treatment. But given the shorter time patients and physicians spend together, the need for specialists in complex cases and the overwhelming levels of therapeutics choices, patients often feel rushed and physicians feel overwhelmed, exhausted, and diminished in their role.

Some physicians and APPs used CPW to deepen their understanding of emotional intelligence, the use of active listening, and the ability to connect through our rounding and support of experiential learning opportunities. A primary tenet of our learning structure was designed with the principles of experiential learning at the center of which is the use of reflection. "Reflection consists of those processes in which learners engage to recapture, notice, and reevaluate their experience, to work with their experience, to turn it into learning."[4] Furthermore, a guiding principle is that "learning does not occur in isolation from social and cultural norms and values."

Experiential learning is reflected in our work with the surgery resident department. The request came to observe and give feedback to the teaching process of surgery residents after observing them in the operating theatre. We observed that faculty relied on shaming in their instruction. For example, faculty could commonly be heard loudly proclaiming, "What are you doing?" when a resident might be in the middle of a complex procedure. And, most often, the faculty would jump in and complete the procedure and complain that the resident had frozen (an expected neurological response to being shouted at under stress and needing to stop and analyze the process in the immediate moment). In a reflection group with faculty and residents after these events, it became clear that this was not an effective learning strategy for several reasons, including initiating "fight-or-flight" neurological functions. The faculty were taught through role-played strategies and then were encouraged to use different instructive interventions. For example, residents might be asked to map out their plan for a procedure before starting. If a concern arose during a procedure, they were to pause and redirect with quiet instruction, such as "Resident A, please pause for a moment; I would like you to do this instead." At the end of the procedure, resident thoughts and feelings were processed, including how they performed, what they learned, and what they would do differently. Faculty and residents both reported the new approach to be less disruptive to the learning environment and that it helped identify areas of deficit without using the cultural norm of shaming.

Using a similar inclusive and respectful questioning approach during COVID-19 has abundantly clarified that we need to rethink the division of labor in providing medical care and the way in which we communicate across specialties and with support staff in all areas of the hospital. Working as a consultant, it was powerful to watch how personnel from different medical and administrative positions, departments, and the community came together quickly, made adjustments to processes, and met a myriad of needs no one had experienced prior to this moment. COVID-19 reminded us that we do not have all the answers and that asking good questions and having respectful dialogue around possible options could bring new awareness and creative solutions. As the people of the world have been attempting to be seen and heard for their individual and cultural contributions for some time, the need to be acknowledged during this pandemic seems to have reached unprecedented levels. That should come as no surprise, since quarantine isolation has led to disconnection in some way for everyone and total isolation for some. Without connection, the act of being affirmed as a valuable person to someone else is missing. In addition, as people are pleading to be seen, heard, and valued, they are ironically more difficult to see as they don masks and protective clothing and are unable to reach out for physical connection. Conversations are more difficult to have through masks, with social distance or through technology, making the discussion of unanswerable questions more difficult to have in good company.

Conclusion: Close the Gaps

"Helping, fixing, and serving represent three different ways of seeing life. When you help, you see life as weak. When you fix, you see life as broken. When you serve, you see life as whole."

~ *Rachel Naomi Remen*

Connection requires one to show up as an integrated person with access to all parts of oneself. My time walking with physicians, APPs, nurses, and all others involved in the delivery of health care impresses upon me that health care itself must become functionally integrated within the current reality, which requires reassessing clinical and professional roles that have undergone so much change as to be unrecognizable and which no longer serve anyone well.

Health care must acknowledge that caring for others requires people to work in functioning multidisciplinary teams where knowing comes from information and experience filtered through emotional intelligence and common sense. When we don't teach people the art of being human and to use all the skills available as humans to communicate, connect, and embrace diversity, when we don't allow those skills to show up at work, everyone is diminished.

When we meet people with the energy and excitement of being on an adventure together, we can serve humanity well. When we connect with others and attempt to see them in their wholeness, we diminish the need to hide parts of ourselves, and we enable all people to venture into the world being truly seen, heard, and valued. Let us start by honoring health care workers by creating a safe environment so they can show us who they really are and what they need in order to do their jobs.

Kathleen Gibney, PhD, LP, ABPP
Psychologist
Consultant

Endnotes

1. Cataldo P, O'Brien D, Byock I. *Palliative Care and Catholic Health Care: Two Millennia of Caring for the Whole Person.* Switzerland: Springer Nature; 2019.

2. Tait S, Jonathan R, Mickey T. Understanding and Addressing Sources of Anxiety Among Health Care Professionals During the COVID-19 Pandemic. *JAMA.* 2020;323(21):2133-2134.

3. Rupp J. *The Cup of Our Life: A Guide for Spiritual Growth.* Notre Dame, IN: Ave Maria Press; 1997.

4. Boud D, Cohen R, Walker D. *Using Experience for Learning.* Buckingham, England: The Society for Research into Higher Education & Open University Press; 1993.

CHAPTER 21

UNLEARNING: FAITH, HUMILITY, AND VULNERABILITY

Carla Park, PhD

Keith Carter, BSc, MD, FRCPC

Physician Case

Dream or reality? My half-asleep brain tries to decide as the feeble vibration of the pager nudges me into consciousness. One eye opens and my brain confirms the page is real. It is another night of "in house" call for CART (COVID Airway Response Team). To ICU stat. I snatch the personal protective equipment (PPE) "go bag" and sprint down the empty hallway, jerking to a stop in front of a sealed-off room. I slow my breathing while putting on layers of PPE: mask, hood, face shield. Peering through the glass, I am relieved to see that the brightly colored, squiggly lines on the monitors are, for the moment, compatible with life.

Once inside my suit of armor against the invisible contagion, I slip through the door and into the red zone. Check and double-check equipment, meds, personnel. The patient's breathing comes in gasps, and the squiggly lines no longer reassure. We have to hurry. Push drugs, breathing stops—that tense moment trying to visualize the airway. Breathing tube in, turn on the ventilator—everything goes well.

My mission is accomplished. Sweat running down the middle of my back, I head out of the red zone. Off with the PPE, hand wash—layer by layer, step by step. As I walk away, the overhead PA system crackles to life: "Code blue, ICU. Code blue, ICU." Wheeling around, I stare at flat lines on the monitor. The code team works frantically inside the bubble. Chest compressions, shock, chest compressions. Then quiet. Another victim of the virus. Another patient I couldn't save. I hang my head in defeat and shuffle down the hallway.

I slink back to my call room and flop onto the cot with body exhausted but mental wheels still spinning. I try escaping into the comforting blackness of unconsciousness, but sleep eludes me. COVID-19 is not the only thing on my mind. My mom is dying from cancer, and we are separated by 3,000 miles and a closed international border. Questions pour into my head like water gushing from a broken faucet, and I can't shut off the tap: "How much time does she have left?" "How can I see her again?" "How will it end?"

Unable to stop the flow, the questions continue, becoming more tangential and philosophical. "How?" switches to "Why?" "Why does it have to be like this?" "Why now?" "Why doesn't God do something?" I heave a weary sigh. "Now I've done it. Brought God into a two-a.m. semiconscious debate on pain and suffering in the world. That should fuel my mental fire and burn up the rest of the night."

Medicine as "Calling" and "Cause"

The reasons for choosing a career in medicine vary, from parent expectations and financial stability to passion for the profession. For some, it rises to the extraordinary sense of a "calling" or even the unmistakable and indescribable urge of a divine calling for a sacred work. The feeling of a calling is often characterized by the sense of a guiding force, purpose, self-fulfillment, personal fit, or altruistic motivation.[1,2]

For this reason, it becomes worth the twelve or more single-focused years ("soul crushing" for some) preparing for it, a career that has, as its primary focus, the relief of suffering.

Not anticipated is that the career might cause suffering, with declining reimbursements, third-party decision makers, and increasing requirements for documentation. Then there is the public health challenge of pandemic, bringing with it longer work hours, inadequate personal protection, new technologies, changing regulations, stressed relationships, social isolation, and conflicting emotions. The current pandemic only highlights the already existing multiple forces that tear at the physician and impinge on the profession—economic, political, financial, and personal. Continued experience of the unknown and emotional tension has its consequences.

Medicine as Burnout

Before COVID-19, approximately 42–44 percent of physicians identified as "feeling burned out"[3] and identified charting and paperwork (bureaucratic tasks) as the number one item related to burnout. With burnout and depression, two-thirds wanted to handle it themselves. They either did not want others to know or felt they could deal with it on their own. In the end, 14 percent reported suicidal thoughts, 1 percent attempted suicide, and 300–400 committed suicide every year (a doctor a day). This results in both negative patient outcomes and negative health outcomes for physicians, not to mention the relative lack of joy related to work. The primary conclusion is that physician burnout is not an individual problem as much as a system or culture problem.

A survey by *Medscape* suggests that the COVID-19 pandemic has only made burnout worse, with two-thirds (64 percent) of United States physicians suggesting that the pandemic has intensified their sense of burnout, with many experiencing an increase in loneliness.[4] Some think about retiring earlier; others think about moving away from the profession itself, resulting in an even greater projected shortfall of physicians by 2025.[5]

Medicine as Humility

What is the antidote? Some suggest that the structure of health care must change, that physicians should have more time to fulfill their capabilities rather than function merely as technicians. While this may be true, the purpose of this paper is to explore the internal structure of the person rather than the environment. A well-known physician scholar gave an address at the opening of a new building at the University of Minnesota as recurrences of a flu pandemic continued. It was 1892, and those who were present listened attentively, not realizing that an even greater pandemic, the pandemic of 1918, was just around the corner. While he began his address as a scholar, William Osler ended it as a preacher, suggesting that, at the end of the day, humility is what matters.[6] He suggested that the physician, more than most, had a sensitivity to personal error and that even the suggestion of a mistake was taken as a slight against personal honor. Speaking against this with the fervor of a preacher, he explored the vulnerability of the physician, suggesting that working with humans would never be an exact science and that the physician must learn to confess errors to self and others, learn from mistakes, and develop a "convenient forgetfulness of our own failings." The physician cannot save every patient or heal every disease, nor can the physician cure the system or erase a pandemic. Sometimes a physician must admit limitations. A modern version of the Hippocratic Oath captures this: "I will remember that there is art to medicine as well as science, and that warmth, sympathy, and understanding may outweigh the surgeon's knife or the chemist's drug. I will not be ashamed to say, 'I know not,' nor will I fail to call in my colleagues when the skills of another are needed for a patient's recovery."[7] Humility, according to Osler, is developed in stillness—"still amidst bustle" and "quiet amidst noise"—and this ability will enable work "for a higher purpose." He encouraged his listeners to appreciate "the fallibility of the faculties upon which you depend . . . and for the sake of what it brings, this grace of humility is a precious gift."[8]

Medicine as Faith

If the physician is the final voice, then where or to whom does the physician turn? One physician identified the need to "shift my gaze" from work to hope, admitting the difficulty of self-generating the hope that is needed.[9] This illustrates the unique connection between humility and faith. It is impossible to admit one's limits if there is not something, someone, or Someone to whom one can turn. Discussions of the similarities between spirituality, faith, and religion are numerous in the literature. The commonalities between the three include searching for a larger life meaning, recognizing a power outside oneself that is higher or transcendent, connectedness, and finally (and most important for the current conversation) is surrendering personal control or admitting that one has a limit, while not being undone by it. There can be strength in vulnerability.

Being a physician is being God-like without being God, having answers without having all the answers, stitching together parts of a story while leaving parts for others to stitch, and journeying with people while also realizing that the destination may change. Selzer, a surgeon and writer, compares doctoring to three things.[10] First, there is a certain "priestliness to the profession," with the doctor taking "vows" (physician oath), wearing regalia (mask and gown), and having a chalice (knife and other instruments). He warns that in being a priest, the physician should not focus on the souls of patients at the expense of letting his/her "own soul lapse" and possibly losing the desire to practice medicine altogether. Second, doctoring is like being a poet, with surgeries and treatments being verses that the poet fashions and through which the physician pours his/her soul. Third, the physician is a traveler in a dangerous country who realizes the perils, seeks at every turn to understand, and travels with others by nature of the profession. These three metaphors—priest, poet, and traveler—capture the complexities of what it means to have humility: to have authority while also not being the authority, to form beauty out of bits and pieces, to travel "with" rather than "in front of," to be a fellow discoverer on journeys of healing.

This is the place of unlearning and of realizing that strength and vulnerability can coexist. Humility is needed, but not the kind that is suggestive of weakness or incompetence. The humility needed has characteristics of unpretentious openness, honest self-disclosure, avoidance of arrogance, and modulation of self-interest.[11] This unlearning—of realizing limits and surrendering personal control—helps bring meaning back into medicine. Humility helps the physician stop, look, and listen, and be

moved by what Osler calls the "poetry of the commonplace"—
the weathered skin of an old man or the bandaged teddy bear of
a wounded child. The physician is vulnerable through his/her
own empathy and compassion.[10] The very struggle not to feel is
the enemy, and humility understands this.

Physician Case Resumes

I know the arguments on both sides. I even know the
broad answers to most of the "why questions." One
thing is certain. Having answers doesn't stop the pain.
I struggle back from the edge of the philosophical abyss
and go back to the practical "how questions": "How
does my relationship with God help/hinder me in times
of intense stress?" "How does my view of God change
the way I cope with pain and anxiety?"

Let's face it. A theoretical God with no connection
to the experiential world is worthless. Indeed, much of
modern society has abandoned the idea of deity because
of this very disconnect. The hurt is real. The fear is real.
The antidote, by necessity, must be real. Is this God
thing real? And if so, how does it all work? How do we
bridge the soul-sucking gap between the theoretical and
experiential?

In my personal life research experiment, I am an
"n=1." Every individual has his/her own unique life lab
environment, complete with criteria and timeline. All I
can do is share the results from my experiment and hope
that the outcome can be reproduced by other people's
research. What have I learned?

The most important breakthrough for me was more
of an unlearning. I came to the realization that there
are situations in life that are simply too hard for me to

cope with. There are situations I am helpless to change, situations where the pain is unbearable. Only when I reach the understanding that there is an actual "end of my rope" am I able to look up and cry out for help.

Conclusion

Currently, there are unfathomable amounts of stress in medicine. Surrendering personal control helps bring meaning back into medicine. At the intersection of medicine, faith, and humility is the concept of unlearning. It is only a partial solution but an important one. Recognition of this will help the profession evolve, not only in the physician's eyes but also in the way care is provided and the way society views the role of the physician as part of a team rather than sole provider. As the physician better understands personal limitation and how it intersects with faith and humility, joy in the practice of medicine will deepen, and patients and communities will increasingly participate in their own care.

Carla Park, PhD
Executive Director, Faith Community Strategy
AdventHealth

Keith Carter, BSc, MD, FRCPC
Anesthesiology/Critical Care
Royal Inland Hospital

Endnotes

1. Yoon JD, Daley BM, Curlin FA. The Association Between a Sense of Calling and Physician Well-Being: A National Study of Primary Care Physicians and Psychiatrists. *Academic Psychiatry.* 2017;41:167-173.

2. Yoon JD, Shin JH, Nian AL, Curlin FA. Religion, Sense of Calling, and the Practice of Medicine: Findings from a National Survey of Primary Care Physicians and Psychiatrists. *Southern Medical Journal.* 2016;108(3):189-195.

3.   Yates SW. Physician Stress and Burnout. *The American Journal of Medicine.* 2019.

4.   Medscape Emergency Medicine Physicians' COVID-19 Experience Report. In. *medscape.com.*

5.   Shanafelt T, Dyrbye L, West C, Sinsky C. Potential Impact of Burnout on the US Physician Workforce. *Mayo Clinic Proceedings.* 2016;91(11):1667-1668.

6.   Osler W, Sir. Teacher and Student. In:1892.

7.   Lasagne. "Would Hippocrates Rewrite His Oath?". In. *The New York Times Magazine*1964:236-239.

8.   Hisae N, Osler W, Sir. *Osler's A Way of Life and Other Addresses, with Commentary and Annotations.* North Carolina: Duke University Press; 2001.

9.   Zacharias R. An Emergency Physician's Spiritual Toolkit to Battle COVID-19. In. *kevinmd.com.* Vol 2020. https://www.kevinmd.com/blog/2020/03/an-emergency-physicians-spiritual-toolkit-to-battle-covid-19.html2020:https://www.kevinmd.com/blog/2020/2003/an-emergency-physicians-spiritual-toolkit-to-battle-covid-2019.html.

10. Selzer R. *Mortal Lessons: Notes on the Art of Surgery.* New York: Simon & Schuster; 1996.

11. Coulehan J. A Gentle and Humane Temper: Humility in Medicine. *Perspectives in Biology and Medicine.* 2011;54(2):206-216.

CHAPTER 22

GETTING TO HEALING: THE CORE OF STORYTELLING IN HEALTH CARE

Martin J. Schreiber, EdD

"The wound is the place where the Light enters you." ~ Rumi[1]

Essence of Healing throughout Life

Healing is an active gesture. We all confront health challenges and ask: How do I get through this? We all face darkness. Healing is a result of conquering the darkness. Life can prepare us for many things, but when it comes to hurt and pain, we never seem prepared. Along the journey, each of us must confront the darkness and move past it, at times navigating through the darkness to reach the light ahead. Or we become paralyzed, alone, stuck, unable to move ahead. Light eludes us.

Voicing our stories and giving reality to our experiences can be particularly liberating to storytellers and invaluable to listeners facing a similar challenge. When one's story is shared with another—a close friend, a coworker, a group of caregivers, or even a public audience—healing often results.

Janine Shepherd was a cross-country skier bound for Olympic greatness when an accident left her paralyzed. As Janine relates in her TED Talk,[2] "A broken body isn't a broken person." She struggled to redefine her identity apart from athletics. She sought to reclaim the power to embrace anything the universe threw at her. "Turn toward the hills," Janine encourages her hearers, "because the magic happens on the other side of the hill. Love the hills. You are resilient." Her story exemplifies the healing influence of storytelling. We all have healing stories just waiting to be shared.

The Healing Stories

In 2018, the podcast *Healing Stories*[3] began a listening narrative approach that takes hearers on a journey into the audio power of story from different leaders in and outside of health care. Each episode features a conversation with a noted leader that illustrates meaningful life lessons. These stories shed light on various ways people respond to difficulties throughout life.

Listening to health care providers offers a powerful glimpse into how physicians address challenges they are confronted with. Here are a few examples as they shared their personal stories:

Life Lessons at the Beginning of a Career

N.C., a family medicine physician,[4] understands the dynamics of living with authenticity. Her interview describes experiences that delve into marriage, self-care, parenting young children, and the complex road of sexuality. N.C. points out that sticking with life along the path can build a world where everyone belongs. She highlights the importance of being authentic and establishing boundaries as critical to her success in dealing with her life experiences.

This early-career physician spoke with ease once her life partner was included in the story. Discerning how to impart comfort and unleash sharing is pivotal. Transparent sharing is dependent upon a sense of safety and trust, creating an opportunity, honesty, and vulnerability.

Life Lessons at Midcareer

P.S., a midcareer cardiologist,[5] shared the importance of a daily practice that involves singing. Born in India and growing up with Catholic education, P.S. admits a need for a consistent thread of resiliency in practice. She leverages her childhood singing connections for strength, endurance, and resilience. Some storytellers escort us to a specific time or moment in their past that carried them through a challenge, disappointment, or loss. Father Jerome Kodell, OSB (the 6th Abbot of Subiaco Abbey),[6] in his book *Life Lessons from the Monastery*, would often say, "You are tripping over the treasure and do not need to go out and search for it in distant lands or libraries." The resources to deal with the challenges that populate our journey may exist within ourselves.

K.W., an internal medicine/pediatric physician,[7] recently traveled to Sondor, Peru, as part of a global health site assessment. During this experience, he reflected on his views of humility, kindness, and meditation. In his words, "A physician transformation means honesty." K.W. is a listening narrator in practice as he invites his patients to tell their story in a typical office visit. He is always listening and responding, "How can I help today?" He listens like a preacher without a pulpit, neither to stand nor judge but as one who releases the patients with freedom to verbalize their experience and, without criticism, to share how they navigated through it.

Moving from room to room every fifteen minutes, he repeats this self-taught approach to patient care. How do we learn to let go of each patient's story as we engage the patient in the next room? It does not have to be difficult. K.W. pauses for 10–15 seconds before going into the room to take a couple of breaths and begin anew; this brief meditation does not have to be lengthy or complex. For in this new room, there will be a new set of challenges, new opportunities to listen and heal.

Life Lessons at End of Career

S.W. is an experienced physician in an Integrative Medicine Program([2]) who loves plants and possesses a profound passion for training family physicians through "continued learning." She asserts that, "Expressing our kindness and unconditional love to each other is the foundation of any relationship that heals." S.W. is forever sharing her wisdom and unlocking her storehouse of experiences for future family physicians. She takes seriously the lives of women in our world, especially those on the margins. Often in the healing stories of the sunset, it is the voice unheard that reenergizes a life passion; S.W. shared her concern, describing women in health care who are often overlooked or neglected. Accurate estimates of the true rate of physician suicide, female or male, may still be lacking, but the risk is not zero and the consequences loom large.[8] How do we create structures for sensitivity and inclusion to turn the tide against exclusivity? As one early-career female physician said, "The entire wall on the way to the lounge is made up of white male physicians. That is not a lounge I want to be at rest in."

S.W. is focused on the perspective of the patient and the ability to listen deeply in her practice of integrating story into the care plan. Her studies provide insights into healing journeys

---

([2]) Dr. Warber retired as a professor at the University of Michigan Department of Family Medicine in 2016. She remains with the department as an active emeritus professor. She is the former co-director of the U-M Integrative Medicine program and was a practicing physician at the Integrative Medicine Clinic located within Briarwood Family Medicine.

by mapping a pattern that involves wisdom and trusted guides along the journey.

Healing in the Midst of a Pandemic

During a *Healing Stories* podcast recorded in 2020 entitled "Life Happens" with Michelle Goetz, MD, the topic of emotion and resilience took center stage.[9] Dr. Goetz, a hospice and palliative care physician, describes herself as a "small town girl." When she is with a patient, she senses the need to take stock of the moment, focus on her breathing and the comfort of her chair, and remind herself of what is real in that moment.

Patients refer to Dr. Goetz's style as one of simply listening: "She talks with me and lets me tell her what I'm going through. It's just nice to have someone to talk to." Dr. Goetz explains, "What palliative care does is try to help patients understand their illnesses."[10]

Dr. Goetz offers a way of seeing today's pandemic through the lens of a rapidly moving train, a "train of emotions" that mimics the feelings her patients experience each day. Imagine as we journey through this crisis, the number of stories to be shared for healing and the true expression of being human.

7 STEPS TO MEANINGFUL STORYTELLING
⊙ Leaders function as listening narrators
⊙ Storytelling helps us see ourselves
⊙ Listen to how others grew from adversity
⊙ Be inclusive and establish a belonging culture
⊙ See those who feel invisible
⊙ Make stories and key actions for growth from stories available
⊙ Develop an Action Playbook for Workforce Resiliency from storytelling

Pope Francis, in his recent book *Let Us Dream*,[11] speaks about the personal crises of our lives. He references the need for us to practice patience and enjoy a healthy sense of humor. He begins *Let Us Dream* by exploring what this crisis can teach us about how to handle upheaval of any kind in our own lives and the world at large. He recalls Friedrich Hölderlin's *Patmos*:[12] "Where the danger is, grows the saving power." At moments of personal trial throughout his life, Pope Francis writes, these words have helped him navigate the crisis. Pope Francis ends with a poem on hope, "Esperanza (Hope)," by Cuban actor and musician Alexis Valdés.

In the practice of medicine, hope informs and infuses our words and our actions. We have all been changed by our experience of the pandemic of 2020, and we are living within a new reality. Hope is an essential element of recovery, resilience, and re-creation.

The practice of storytelling has the capacity to contribute to our healing, make us more resilient, enrich our relationships, build community, and fulfill our mission. I'm listening. Tell me your story.

Martin J. Schreiber, EdD
Vice President, Mission Leadership Institute
Providence St. Joseph Health

Endnotes

1. Rumi Ja-D. *The Essential Rumi.* Harper and Row - Books; 1995.

2. Shepherd J. A Broken Body Isn't A Broken Person [Internet]: Ted. com; 2012. Podcast. Available from: https://www.ted.com/talks/janine_shepherd_a_broken_body_isn_t_a_broken_person?language=en

3. Schreiber MJ. Healing Stories [Internet]: Apple.com; 2020. Podcast. Available from: https://podcasts.apple.com/us/podcast/healing-stories/id1364307287

4. Groeschl MD N. Dancing Through Life with Dr. Nicole Groeschl, MD [Internet]:Apple.com;2018.Podcast.Availablefrom:https://podcasts.apple. com/us/podcast/dancing-through-life-with-dr-nicole-groeschl-md/id1364307287?i=1000467096866

5. Sanon MD P. Dr. Priyanka Sanon; A Physician is Never Alone [Internet]: Apple.com; 2018. Podcast. Available from: https://podcasts.apple. com/us/podcast/dr-priyanka-sanon-a-physician-is-never-alone/id1364307287?i=1000413259211

6. Kodell J. *Life Lessons from the Monastery : Wisdom on Love, Prayer, Calling, and Commitment.* Word Among Us Press; 2010.

7. Wagner MD K. Dr. Kendall Wagner M.D., A Physician transformation means honesty [Internet]: Apple.com; 2018. Podcast. Available from: https://podcasts.apple.com/us/podcast/dr-kendall-wagner-m-d-physician-transformation-means/id1364307287?i=1000417056945

8. Gold K, Schwenk T. Physician Suicide-A Personal and Community Tragedy. *JAMA Psychiatry.* 2020;77(6):559-560.

9. Goetz M. Life Happens with Dr. Michelle Goetz [Internet]. Podcast. Available from: https://podcasts.apple.com/us/podcast/ life-happens-with-dr-michelle-goetz/id1364307287

10. Cernich K. 'Slow Medicine' - Palliative Care Offers Support, Comfort for Patients with Serious Illnesses. 2020. https://www.emissourian.com/ features_people/feature_stories/slow-medicine-palliative-care-offers-support-comfort-for-patients-with-serious-illnesses/article_30809cd8-2e6a-11ea-8c67-f3ab973d095e.html.

11. PopeFrancis, Ivereigh A. *Let Us Dream: The Path to a Better Future.* New York, NY USA: Simon & Schuster; 2020.

12. Patmos. Vers 3f. in: Gedichte von Friedrich Hölderlin, Druck und Verlag von Philipp Reclam jun., Leipzig 1873, S. 133. https://quotepark.com/ quotes/720168-friedrich-holderlin-but-where-the-danger-is-also-grows-the-saving-pow/. Published 1803. Accessed.

CHAPTER 23

RESILIENCE, STORYTELLING, AND CARING FOR OTHERS: AN INTERSECTION

Martin J. Schreiber, EdD

"Life isn't about waiting for the storm to pass. It's about learning how to dance in the rain."[1] ~ *Vivian Greene*

Introduction

Today's transformation of health care is progressing at an unimaginable pace. New electronic technologies, the intense shift to value-based care, cultural shifts in providers and patient populations, and the unrelenting focus on cost and efficiency have assumed center stage, all contributing to a system and health care profession in flux. This trend is expected to continue as health care leaders are guiding hospital networks and health systems at a time when natural disasters, social unrest, and worldwide pandemics are disrupting the historic operational framework for success.

These events result in incalculable stressors which lead to physician burnout,[2] an impending nursing shortage,[3] and fewer graduates pursuing a career in health care–related fields. We cannot wait for this apparent storm confronting the United States health care system to pass, but rather, as leaders, we need to focus on how we can bring all members of the organization together today. As John Kennedy declared in a speech that was prepared for delivery in Dallas in 1963,[4] "Leadership and learning are indispensable to each other." If we expect to lead others through stormy times like today in health care, we must continue to learn about ourselves and from others, especially as we all navigate through life's adversities.

In the midst of the current health care storm lives the realization that health care professionals are not alone in what life teaches all of us about caring for others. The passion for caring begins with truly "seeing" each individual working in a health care setting as a unique person in the healing quest of medicine. Preserving the "human touch of caring" amid an ever-changing world is at the core of creating a successful care model for the future. Safeguarding the human connections in this new delivery model will depend on galvanizing an extremely stressed health care workforce to focus on treating patients as people.[5] This highly focused commitment will require a tighter working relationship between all sectors of the health care delivery system. Storytelling built upon life experiences can be a valuable tool as organizations seek to build resiliency in the workforce.

The current chapter will examine where storytellers come from, look into the art of storytelling from Homer to Murrow, examine the varied types of storytelling, and outline steps that nurture the storytelling exercise for health care organizations.

Leadership, Purpose, and Future Success

As with any traumatic experience, what matters is how we continually learn about ourselves as we adapt and grow from individual challenges. What we learn is that it's not just about whether we succeed or fail, but rather how we, as individuals, grow from our challenges to not only enhance individual resilience, but that of our families and our workplace. When we think about health care delivery and the legions of people involved in ensuring every patient's experience, "everyone belongs," and every individual plays a critical role in achieving a differentiated experience through voicing their individual life lesson.

The collection artwork that hangs in the hall of Cleveland Clinic's Miller Family Heart, Vascular & Thoracic Institute (Illustration 1) reminds all who enter that the fabric of every organization not only consists of people who are highly visible but also those who contribute behind the scenes and below the surface.

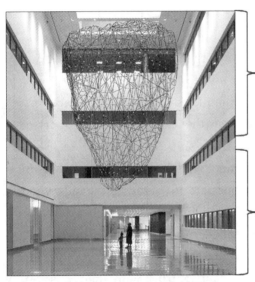

IÑIGO MANGLANO-OVALLE (B. SPAIN) BLUEBERG
(R11I01), 2007 SUSPENDED ANODIZED ALUMINUM.
PHOTO USED BY PERMISSION OF CLEVELAND CLINIC.

Physicians, nurses,
non-physician
practitioners
CEO, COO, CMO, CNO,
CFO, Mission Leaders
Administrative/front desk

Dietary/food service
workers
Environmental service
workers
Lab personnel
Rehabilitation Services
Radiology personnel
Finance/Billing
Security/Safety
Pharmacy
Parking/transportation
workers
IT/ Records/Compliance/
Legal

Illustration 1

The 30-foot-tall hanging sculpture is seen by thousands of people each day. Manglano-Ovalle collaborated with many partners, including scientists and engineers, to create BlueBerg (r11i01). He refers to the work as "a structure of support. And I think that's a good metaphor not only for Cleveland Clinic but also for the human body when it should be in a healthy state." The fabric of every organization consists of many caregivers, those the patient sees, but so many more that are never seen. Taken together, the total care structure gives life to the patient experience and maintains the health of any organization just like the human body.

More than anything else, people, not cash and capital goods, are what make up an organization. When large-scale change arrives, everyone is affected, and leaders play a key role in bringing people together. Leaders make sure that every team member knows that they themselves are a key part of successful change, and the leadership team is there to listen, provide valuable encouragement, and define everyone's role. In change, everyone plays a major part. An organization fails when it's exclusive, when it develops a myopic approach to driving difficult change, or forgets that every transition is not successful. Organizations are at risk when they do not incorporate life lessons from those they hire and entrust with their mission. However, by leveraging the life stories that diverse workers across the delivery network have experienced, leaders can enhance an organization's resilience and chances for success. There is wisdom in listening to others.

The poet William Stafford writes of the manner in which human adaptation to life experience weaves a thread that stabilizes one's life journey.[6] We have the opportunity to learn and grow as we face each new challenge. And our stories of patience and perseverance can prove invaluable to others along the way.

The Art of Storytelling

Storytelling is important in all cultures to not only hear but also to tell. Every story serves a purpose, even if to simply relay a message. The earliest form of storytelling that has been discovered is from the Lascaux Caves in the Pyrenees Mountains[7] in southern France from between 15,000 and 13,000 BC depicting a variety of animals and one image of a human being. Advancing some 10,000 years, the "Epic of Gilgamesh" is considered one of the great literary masterpieces of ancient times, followed in 700 BC by Homer's story of Odysseus's journey returning to the island of Troy. Over the next several centuries, the art of the written word and storytelling would evolve and develop into cohesive works, like the Bible and the multiple works of William Shakespeare. Today, we tell stories through multiple methods of illustrations, written word, oral storytelling, digital websites, and podcasts.

There is an art to storytelling, and the role of being the listening narrator brings the most out of the person telling the story. Ira Glass,[8] the executive producer of *This American Life*, created a platform through National Public Radio (NPR) to center on value-loaded lessons from the most basic form of storytelling: the anecdote. Glass keeps us engaged by throwing out questions to keep his audience listening, creating tension by the unanswered question. He enables the storyteller to be free, without a judgment, to say what they desire to say. There is much to be learned from tuning in to *This American Life*.

The radio hour *The Moth*[9] highlights the art and craft of storytelling, featuring prominent literary and cultural personalities who speak facing a live audience about real things that have happened to them. Another example of podcast storytelling is *StoryCorps*,[10] a creative approach of engaging people to tell their story in the "safe space" of a phone booth setting.

During its four years on NPR, *This I Believe*[11] engaged listeners in a discussion of core beliefs that guide daily life. Beginning in 1951 with Edward R. Murrow hosting, the listening audience heard from people in all walks of life: the very young and the very old, the famous and the previously unknown, Nobel laureates, teachers, prison inmates, students, politicians, farmers, poets, entrepreneurs, activists, and executives. Sharing life lessons proved to be a poignant approach for listeners, learning through the storyteller's personal lens on life.

Videos are also storytelling tools that impact how we interpret life situations, and we sometimes find they are very different than they appear at first glance. The award-winning video by the Cleveland Clinic on empathy[12] unveiled the truest meaning to the words, "If you could stand in someone else's shoes . . . Hear what they hear. See what they see. Feel what they feel. Would you treat them differently?" When we relate to those around us by understanding their individual stories and circumstances, we improve the way we work, the way we live our lives, the way we care for one another, and the way we relate to one another. Empathy connects us to one other.

The Storyteller, Life's Challenges, and Sharing

Lisa Pocius, MD, in the book *Surfing the Sea of Change*, examines the essence of adapting to life's traumas when she noted that someone who is resilient is someone who grows. We don't handle a situation the same way each time we are confronted with a challenge. Hopefully, each response builds on experiences from the past as we grow and adapt. Learning from the past and getting better at handling change is certainly a "skill that has to be developed and practiced." You don't have to be famous to have an impact on people; it's about your life story. Every story matters.

Practical approaches to getting comfortable with telling one's story[13] include the following:

1. A recognition of the value of diversity. Inclusivity, dignity, and respect are foundational components to mission and culture. Storytellers come from all corners of the health care delivery system. Inclusivity is key.[14]
2. Comfort with telling one's story requires a sense of "psychological safety." A Google study, "Project Aristotle," recognizes psychological safety as the key element of a high-performing team.[15]
3. Becoming a listening narrator is critically important for storytelling success. Just listen. It is critical not to interrupt people telling their story. This reverence, attention, and devotion for the story is an essential component of freedom in relating lessons learned.[16]
4. Affirming the storyteller as the narrative progresses is often helpful to those dealing with crisis, trauma, or change.
5. Engage the storyteller's summary of learning from life experience.

A listening narrative approach to conducting the interview assists in clarifying the lesson from the experience by not questioning or judging the message. It is critical to give the storyteller the comfort and freedom to share personal experience with a transparency that allows for a distinct humanness in the act of sharing. Every story has a beginning, a middle, and an end; the critical nature of storytelling is capturing how growth occurred and adaption took place, with the narrator as the lamplighter guiding the way.

As noted by the author and motivational speaker Simon Sinek, in his book *Start With Why*,[17] leaders who've had the greatest influence in the world all think, act, and communicate the same way. They inspire cooperation, trust, and change by positioning the "why" at the center of how we lead; success is achieved through focusing on driving change from within. Our "why" is driving how we see a challenge, how we move forward with optimism for success. Our "why" provides a framework upon which organizations can be built, movements can be led, and people can be inspired. So sharing is powerful, and we can make a difference by telling our story.

Conclusion

The next decade will require a focus on the true belief that every individual's life story matters, and the essence of a system or an organization's culture rests within the realization that in sharing lessons from life experiences resides a special inclusivity and commitment to caring for all. Success in health care starts with people feeling they belong, a realization that multicultural backgrounds bring a richness to the fabric of all organizations. As leaders, we need to provide opportunities for storytelling and construct the stage for all to share lessons learned, illuminate the adaptions that were made, and acquire that growth necessary to conquer future challenges.

As we champion a storytelling approach to galvanizing a health care team, individuals will become more resilient and organizations healthier.

Martin J. Schreiber, EdD
Vice President, Mission Leadership Institute
Providence St. Joseph Health

Endnotes

1. Green V. Dance Your Dance. In: *Believe You Can Fly!*: Blurb; 2013: https://www.blurb.com/b/2904265-dance-your-dance?ebook=381076.

2. Hartzband P, Groopman J. Physician Burnout, Interrupted. *New England Journal of Medicine*. 2020;382(26):2485-2487.

3. U.S. Department of Health and Human Services HRaSA, Analysis NCfHW. The Future of the Nursing Workforce: National- and State-Level Projections, 2012-2025. In. Rockville, Maryland, USA2014.

4. Kennedy JF. Remarks Prepared for Delivery at the Trade Mart in Dallas, TX, November 22, 1963 [Undelivered]1963.

5. Lalanda M, Gracia-Peligero E, DelgadoMarroquín M. They Are People First, Then Patients. *AMA Journal of Ethics*. 2017;19(5):508-509.

6. Stafford W. *The Way It Is: New and Selected Poems*. Graywolf Press; 1999.

7. Ruspoli M. *The Cave of Lascaux: The Final Photographs*. Publisher: Harry N. Abrams; 1987.

8. Glass I. Ira Glass on Storytelling. In: thisamericanlife.org; 2009.

9. Burns C, Gopnik A, Green G. *The Moth*. Hachette Books; 2013.

10. Isay D. *Ties That Bind: Stories of Love and Gratitude from the First Ten Years of StoryCorps*. New York USA: Penguin Group; 2014.

11. Allison J. *This I Believe : the Personal Philosophies of Remarkable Men and Women*. New York, USA: Henry Holt and Company LLC; 2006.

12. Gillis TT. Empathy [Internet]: onbeing.org; 2013. Podcast. Available from: https://onbeing.org/blog/an-empathy-video-that-asks-you-to-stand-in-someone-elses-shoes/

13. Dunne J. How to Build a Culture of Resilience at Your Organization. In. *Virgin Pulse.com* 2020.

14. Rohr R. *Falling Upward : A Spirituality for the Two Halves of Life.* San Francisco, CA USA: Jossey-Bass; 2011.

15. Bariso J. After Years of Research, Google Discovered the Secret Weapon to Building a Great Team. It's a Lesson in Emotional Intelligence. Years of research provide a major clue as to how to get the most out of your team. *Inccom.* 2020. https://www.inc.com/justin-bariso/after-years-of-research-google-discovered-secret-weapon-to-building-a-great-team-its-a-lesson-in-emotional-intelligence.html.

16. Gray H. Ignatian Spirituality: What are We Talking about and Why?2002, SaintPeters.edu.

17. Sinek S. *Start with Why: How Great Leaders Inspire Everyone to Take Action.* New York, NY, USA: Penguin Group; 2011.

CHAPTER 24

COMPASSION ROUNDS: CARING FOR PARENTS OF OUR TINIEST NEWBORNS

Jocelyn Shaw, MDiv

Reina Mayor, MD

Introduction

Compassion Rounds (CR) is a collaboration between physician and chaplain to better serve the psychosocial, emotional, and spiritual needs of the parents to the patients in the neonatal intensive care unit (NICU). The unique style of rounds requires attention to details and processes that are unique to health care in style and approach. The benefits not only impact our patients and families but simultaneously show great positive reward to the health care members who are engaged through the process.

Why Were Compassion Rounds Established?

Compassion Rounds were created as a partnership between the physician and the chaplain to communicate with the patient and family utilizing a psychosocial, emotional, and spiritual approach to medical care. Compassion Rounds were established within AdventHealth for the children's neonatal intensive care unit after adopting the concept from Dr. John Guarneri, who previously used a similar method in the adult areas of the hospital. From a physician's perspective, I was interested in participating in CR but uncertain how it would fit into our busy NICU schedule. On our first day of CR, I was having classic symptoms of physician burnout. I was coming off an intense service block that had taken its toll on me physically and emotionally. I was surprised how I was immediately drawn to the mothers' stories. My exhaustion was quickly forgotten as I sat there and listened to moms detail their concerns and struggles. I had spent three weeks speaking with these moms on a daily basis about their infants' medical conditions yet had no idea that they were silently suffering.

My experience with CR continues to be personally uplifting. It has been very rewarding to give my time to listen to moms, validate their struggles, and encourage them. The spiritual aspect of CR involving prayer has had the most profound impact on my well-being as a person and a physician. The burden of caring for critically ill infants at times can seem unsurmountable. Standing together holding hands, surrounding a baby's Isolette®, and praying together as a unified team is powerful and helps lift the burden that I carry as a physician. I often refer to CR as "chicken soup for a physician's soul."

Over the course of the past few years of conducting CR, Jocelyn and I have identified many moms struggling with postpartum depression and anxiety. The time that follows a NICU admission is "unnatural" and filled with many changes and struggles for the mother specifically. The NICU environment, infant's appearance, difficulties bonding, separation from baby, loss of parental role, spiritual upheaval, guilt for not carrying to term, and symptoms of postpartum depression are among the many reasons that NICU moms have increased risk of anxiety. In a study by Lefkowitz et al., 35 percent of mothers met the criteria for acute stress disorder after five days of NICU admission, and 15 percent met diagnostic for post-traumatic stress disorder after 30 days of the NICU admission.[1] It is not surprising that postpartum depression (PPD) is the most common medical problem a new mother will face, and mothers of preterm infants are twice as likely to experience PPD than women who deliver full-term infants.[2-5]

CR identified a significant gap in care for the parents/families of our NICU babies. We were thoroughly addressing the infants' medical needs but not addressing maternal well-being, which can impair maternal-infant interactions, leading to poor bonding, developmental delay, and social interaction difficulties in affected children.[6] As many as 46 percent of women who experience PPD symptoms continue to have symptoms one year after the birth of their child.[6] It should be noted that while CR was created in the NICU working with postpartum parents, physicians and chaplains are caring for critically ill patients and families who frequently experience increased depression and anxiety.

Purpose of Compassion Rounds

The purpose for CR is to provide a safe place for parents/families to receive emotional and spiritual care. As the physician leads the interdisciplinary team's efforts, the chaplain works in tandem with the physician. The chaplain's role is to come alongside and partner with the physician and team to focus on the emotional and spiritual care of the family. The CR session creates a sacred place where the group can journey together for a designated time to assist the families in finding hope, strength, and peace. During this time of exploration and support, the CR team seeks to empower the families to uncover ways of coping. Consequently, finding new paths of coping will also improve the maternal well-being and strengthen the infant-mother bond.[6] Spiritual care has been shown to help overall health and bolster the ability of individuals to cope with difficulties. "On examining the relationship between spirituality and health, it has been observed that spirituality helps to prevent disease, improve health, and facilitate coping with difficulties."[7-9]

What Compassion Rounds Are in Practice and How They Differ from Medical Rounds

Integral to the success of CR, the physician and chaplain must take time to develop a working relationship with one another. A strong trust between the chaplain and doctor is the key. The sacred place explored in the patient's journey is one of intimacy, and for this to take place organically, the chaplain and physician must have a true partnership and trust built prior to beginning this work.

For the NICU team at AdventHealth for Children, the scheduled service blocks for physicians is based on a three-week rotation. Therefore, planning a one- or two-hour session for CR works well when scheduled once per month. This schedule allows room for the physician to get to know their patients by the end of the service block and for the chaplain to partner with them as they ascertain which patients might benefit the most from these rounds. Due to time constraints, only four to five families are offered CR each month. Since it is often not obvious which patients are the most in need of CR, educational information is provided in each NICU room inviting all NICU families to participate in CR. However, we have found that most families do not actively seek out CR unless the chaplain or physician personally speaks with them directly about the process. Thus, in our institution, the high-risk families are identified by the medical team and offered CR. Social workers and nurse leaders for the unit also help in identifying the families that might best be served by this type of support.

Once families are identified, the chaplain then works with the families, allowing time for them to ask questions and gauging if CR interests them. As the chaplain engages with the families, they are able to see that CR is different from the daily multidisciplinary rounds that they have experienced; the focus is not on the medical aspects but on the psychosocial, emotional, and spiritual support they need. This is a significant shift in focus that centers around how the parents are coping. Prior to CR, the chaplain will connect with the families to ensure they are available to meet with the doctor and confirm participation. Each family is given approximately 20–30 minutes for their CR.

The day of the CR, the session begins with the doctor offering a brief overview of the patient's hospital stay with the team. The team enters the room, and the doctor introduces each attendee. CR may include a social worker, nurse practitioner, family care consultant, nurse, and a child life specialist. CR is most effective if it involves a maximum of only four people or fewer; at minimum, the physician and chaplain must be present.

The physician then intentionally describes the ground rules for the session; primarily, medicine will not be discussed. We do not discuss test results or the medical plan of care. This establishes a safe space for families. Families of critically ill patients live in a constant state of bracing themselves for more bad news.

At the start of CR, the physician often says, "During medical rounds, we discuss in detail the medical plan of care. However, we often do not have an opportunity to find out how you are doing and how you are coping. CR provides an opportunity for us to learn more about how you are." The chaplain then follows with further context by sharing, "Compassion Rounds is a time for key interdisciplinary team members to come and sit with you to understand and be a part of your journey and build support for you. It gives us a chance to understand your context and what is important to you." Following this, the physician and chaplain engage with real-time open-ended questions to invite the parents to share openly about their journey. Please note that chaplains typically use spiritual assessments to guide their pastoral intervention process during CR by utilizing a conversational approach.[10]

Learnings from Compassion Rounds

During the three and a half years that CR have been a part of the NICU experience, a few things have been noted. It is key that the chaplain engage the family ahead of time. Often, the family does not understand the role of the chaplain in general or as a part of these rounds. This puts the family at ease and educates them about the integral role of the chaplain. This step is imperative, and the chaplain takes the lead connecting with families prior to the rounds. The connection also provides context and education for the family while simultaneously building rapport. AdventHealth extends a unique health care approach that utilizes the chaplain as an "opt-out" versus an "opt-in" method. Essentially, the chaplain is considered a key part of the care team, and this is clearly demonstrated during CR, as the chaplain plays the role of the physician's right hand in partnering and navigating through the whole-care approach to the patient's needs. This symbiotic relationship between the physician and the chaplain is also illustrated by how both parties work together to provide whole-person care to the family during this unique style of rounds.

The family is accustomed to seeing the physician as the leader in medical rounds when medicine and care plans are discussed, but during CR, the focus is not on medicine. The chaplain seeks to find commonalities between patients and the care team.[11] Members of the team use the time to check in on the parents' emotional and spiritual well-being since not much time is allotted for this during medical rounds. Therefore, CR provides an established, safe space for the family to share and engage coping skills with members of the interdisciplinary team, with the primary emphasis on the psychosocial, emotional, and spiritual support measures. Typically, medical professionals must focus on the medical conditions; however, CR invites the interdisciplinary team into more of the chaplain's area of work that seeks to understand the person as a whole.[12]

Personal Perspective from the Collaborating Chaplain and Co-Creator

After one of the first CRs was hosted, I remember turning to Dr. Mayor and hearing her share how CR had reconnected her to her passion for medicine. I recall her saying, "This is why I went into medicine." After spending the day deep in the trenches of the work I am so passionate about and hearing the doctor that I admire share how passionate she was for this collaboration, I was sold! I thought, "I'm in!" If AdventHealth and chaplain ministry had not completely won me over already, I was convinced in this moment that I was fully dedicated to this calling. As this CR journey unfolded, I felt invested in a work that was much larger than myself, and I was so grateful to be a part of this journey. What grew out of CR for me was a passion to continue to collaborate with physicians and team members. Another opportunity I saw evolving over the course of the rounds was a unique building of trust between the doctors and the parents. The parents saw the doctors in a new light. The doctor was able, within the emotional space created, to show their own empathy for each person as who they are—a mother, a father, a person. It was not that the doctor did not care prior to the inception of CR, but this time allowed for the parents to see the physician demonstrating, through conversation and time, how much they care for them by their simple presence. For me to be a part of this process and contribute, from my professional perspective, has been an inestimable honor.

Jocelyn Shaw, MDiv
Senior Chaplain
AdventHealth for Children

Reina Mayor, MD
Neonatology
AdventHealth Orlando

Endnotes

1. Lefkowitz DS, Baxt C, Evans JR. Prevalence and Correlates of Posttraumatic Stress and Postpartum Depression in Parents of Infants in the Neonatal Intensive Care Unit (NICU). *Journal of Clinical Psychology in Medical Settings.* 2010;17(3):230-237.

2. Wisner K, Parry B, Piontek C. Clinical Practice. Postpartum Depression. *The New England Journal of Medicine.* 2002;347(3):194-199.

3. Gennaro S. Postpartal Anxiety and Depression in Mothers of Term and Preterm Infants. *Nursing Research.* 1988;37(2):82-85.

4. Logsdon MC, Davis DW, Wilkerson SA, Birkimer JC. Predictors of Depression in Mothers of Preterm Infants. *Journal of Social Behavior and Personality.* 1997;12(1):73-88.

5. Gönülal D, Yalaz M, Altun-Köroğlu O, Kültürsay N. Both Parents of Neonatal Intensive Care Unit Patients Are at Risk of Depression. *The Turkish Journal of Pediatrics.* 2014;56(2):171-176.

6. Beck C. The Effects of Postpartum Depression on Child Development: A Meta-Analysis. *Archives of Psychiatric Nursing.* 1998;12(1):12-20.

7. Dilek KA, Funda KÖ, Fatma GT. The Effect of Spiritual Care on Stress Levels of Mothers in NICU. *Western Journal of Nursing Research.* 2018;40(7):997-1011.

8. Modjarrad K. Medicine and Spirituality. *Journal of the American Medical Association.* 2004;291(23):2880.

9. Wilson S, Miles M. Spirituality in African-American Mothers Coping with a Seriously Ill Infant. *Journal of the Society of Pediatric Nurses : JSPN.* 2001;6(3):116-122.

10. Lewis JM. Pastoral Assessment in Hospital Ministry: A Conversational Approach. *Chaplaincy Today.* 2002;18(2):5-13.

11. Cadge W, Sigalow E. Negotiating Religious Differences: The Strategies of Interfaith Chaplains in Healthcare: INTERFAITH CHAPLAINS IN HEALTHCARE. *Journal for the Scientific Study of Religion.* 2013;52(1):146-158.

12. de Vries R, Berlinger N, Cadge W. Lost in Translation: The Chaplain's Role in Health Care. *The Hastings Center Report.* 2008;38(6):23-27.

CHAPTER 25

SCREENING FOR SPIRITUAL WHOLENESS: ADVENTHEALTH'S CLINICAL MISSION INTEGRATION PROGRAM

The following article originally appeared in the September 2020 issue of *Healthcare Business Insights, part of Clarivate*. It is reprinted by permission of the publisher.

What Does It Mean?

Spiritual wellness can have a profound impact on one's overall physical health but is often overlooked in the fast-paced healthcare setting. Recognizing spirituality as an integral part of whole-person care, leaders at AdventHealth developed a program that incorporates a spiritual wholeness screening into both the inpatient and outpatient care. By asking patients three targeted questions, the organization is able to identify unmet spiritual and social needs. Since its inception in 2018, AdventHealth's clinical mission integration program has screened more than five million patients across the system, generating more than 20,000 referrals for spiritual services.

Recent literature demonstrates an association between spiritual wellness practices (such as prayer, religious counseling, and church attendance) and physical health. While more conclusive research is needed, some past studies have suggested spiritual wellness practices may be beneficial to quality of life and management of chronic diseases such as hypertension, coronary artery disease, HIV/AIDS, and diabetes mellitus, as explored in a 2017 systematic review published in *PLoS One*. Despite this, spirituality is sometimes considered a controversial topic in the clinical setting, and, as a result, patients' spiritual needs can go unaddressed. AdventHealth, a nonprofit faith-based healthcare system headquartered in Altamonte Springs, Florida, sought to change that narrative. To do this, leadership developed a comprehensive clinical mission integration program to harmonize the clinical and spiritual aspects of patient care.

"We wanted to get to the core of spiritual-emotional issues without saying, 'Now we're going to take the spiritual-emotional history,'" said Ted Hamilton, MD, chief mission integration officer and senior vice president of mission and ministry for AdventHealth. "On an average day in AdventHealth, we'll admit 1,000 patients across our hospitals. In the outpatient setting, we may see as many as 20,000 patients. So, in a year's time, we can touch as many as four or five million patients with these spiritual wholeness questions."

Building the Case and Obtaining Buy-In

AdventHealth's journey toward what is now its spiritual wholeness screening began in 2013. Collaborating with researchers at Duke University, the organization conducted a study to assess the willingness of system clinicians to embrace spiritual practices in the outpatient setting. In a 12-month intensive educational training program, nearly 450 AdventHealth clinicians were provided the training, resources, and tools to engage in spiritual practices with their patients. Practices included clinician-led prayer, self-disclosure of religious beliefs, encouragement of patients' religious beliefs, and chaplain referral.

The study demonstrated significant changes in clinician behavior as a result of the training, including an increase in the frequency of clinicians praying with patients as well as the frequency of chaplain referral. Four papers were published in peer-reviewed medical literature with their findings, and the team was able to demonstrate the rigor behind the program as well as the willingness of clinicians—and patients—to embrace spiritual practices.

Encouraged by the results of their preliminary research, the AdventHealth team visited Mercy Hospital St. Louis, a faith-based healthcare system that had successfully implemented a similar program over several years. Gleaning insights from the achievements of a comparable program, the team was equipped to build a powerful business case for the executive leadership team at AdventHealth. With the support of leadership, the program was able to secure the necessary resources to create a comprehensive clinical mission integration program and now invests $5 million in the program annually.

Clinical Mission Integration Program Rollout Program Resources

In 2018, AdventHealth hired 38 clinical mission integration specialists as well as a program director and program assistant. The clinical mission integration specialists were responsible for engaging with the employed physician groups throughout the system. Over about a six-month period, these specialists facilitated the integration of spiritual care practices throughout the entire outpatient network. By late 2019, the program was being rolled out across AdventHealth's inpatient network as well.

The organization also established a call center (the "e-spiritual care center") at the corporate headquarters staffed by trained spiritual caregivers. Three full-time caregivers staff the call center, with four to five PRN caregivers available as needed.

Examples of Support Provided by Spiritual Caregivers at AdventHealth

- ⊙ Conducting spiritual needs assessments
- ⊙ Creating individualized spiritual care plans
- ⊙ Providing spiritual counseling
- ⊙ Praying with patients
- ⊙ Reading holy scriptures with patients
- ⊙ Providing religious resources, such as inspirational readings or texts
- ⊙ Connecting patients with community resources, such as social services or local churches

Spiritual Wholeness Screening

A three-question spiritual wholeness screening tool was developed by the clinical mission integration team. Focusing on the key "spiritual indicators" of love, joy, and peace, the questionnaire was designed to assess the patient's spiritual-emotional condition. The tool is administered to all patients willing to answer the questions at intake in both the outpatient and inpatient settings. Responses are then integrated into the patient's electronic health record. Screening questions are:

- ⊙ Do you have someone who loves and cares for you?
- ⊙ Do you have a source of joy in your life?
- ⊙ Do you have a sense of peace today?

In the inpatient setting, if a patient answers "no" to any of the spiritual wholeness questions, the system triggers an automatic referral to one of the hospital's chaplains. The chaplain will then follow up with the patient to provide spiritual support while the patient is in the hospital.

In the outpatient setting, if a patient answers "no" to any of the spiritual wholeness questions, the physician is notified. The care team can either address the issue during the patient's visit or, if additional resources are required, place a referral to the e-spiritual care center. A spiritual caregiver receives the referral, contacts the patient, and then sends a consultation report to the physician, which also becomes part of the patient's record.

The e-spiritual care center staff will contact the patient up to three times to provide spiritual support. While the primary goal is to provide spiritual support for patients, the center serves secondarily as an information hub that can also connect patients with resources in their community, based on the identified need. This could include social services, community churches, or even local AdventHealth chaplains.

Educating Staff

The clinical mission integration specialists underwent an intensive initial training program, followed by quarterly continuing education sessions. Specialists regularly visit physician offices throughout the system to provide educational tools, resources, and support to frontline staff. These tools include presentations from leadership, workshops on physician engagement and wellness, and training on spiritual care.

"Very quickly, the specialists became a resource to the physician offices during their visits," Hamilton said. "It was not unusual for a staff member to ask, 'Could you spend a few minutes with me before you go?' and they'd step back to a private place and say, 'I'm facing a divorce and it's hard for me to keep my mind on work. Would you pray with me?' What was intended to be a resource for patients ended up indirectly being very valuable to staff and physicians, too."

Program Results

AdventHealth's clinical mission integration program has screened more than five million patients across the system, generating more than 20,000 referrals for spiritual services. While it can be a challenge to measure spiritual wholeness, the e-spiritual care center records "mission moments," or standout interactions with patients whose lives were touched in a positive way by the program. Since its inception, AdventHealth's clinical mission integration program has recorded over 1,000 of these "mission moments," demonstrating the program's far-reaching impact. Patients and staff alike have responded positively to the program, which reflects the organization's deep commitment to whole-person care.

Healthcare Business Insights, part of Clarivate

Editor's Addendum

Ted Hamilton, MD, MBA

One might ask how the topic of Spiritual Wholeness Screening (SWS) is relevant to physician well-being. Currently, over 1,600 AdventHealth physicians and advanced practice providers incorporate Spiritual Wholeness Screening into their practices, generating 80–100 patient referrals daily to the AdventHealth e-spiritual care center.

A few random comments from participating providers reveal a sense of the satisfaction that both patients and caregivers experience:

"The spiritual wholeness questions lead patients to be more open, and they know from the beginning of the visit that we care about the way they feel." ~ Marva Marcius, NP

"Spiritual health is of utmost importance in my line of work. I treat in the spirit of love, peace, kindness, gentleness, and self-control to the best of my ability." ~ Holly Marie Lindberg, MD

"The reaction has been nothing short of amazing. Praying brings tears to many and deep gratitude to others. Everyone thanks me. I feel blessed to bring them comfort." ~ Cal Fischer, DO

"Screening our patients opens a door to our patients' lives beyond our office. I am treating them for a medical condition but caring about them mind, body, and spirit." ~ Brittany Garrett, APRN

"Taking time to pray with a patient. . . often provides greater healing than any medical treatment or advice I can offer them." ~ Shea Humphrey, DO

"It is a blessing when I can treat the entire patient in the family practice setting—physical, emotional, and spiritual. It speaks of a higher love and care that goes beyond the human factor." ~ Valorie Mixon, PAC

These brief reflections from practicing clinicians are indicative of the experiences of many—patient interactions characterized by increased openness, transparency, appreciation, and richer, deeper relationships between patients and caregivers contributing to greater fulfillment in the practice of medicine.

CHAPTER 26

THE WHOLE CLINICIAN: INTEGRATING SPIRITUALITY AND PRACTICE

John C. Welch, PhD

Medical Care amid the Pandemic

Of several countries across the globe, the United States was one whose citizens began battling COVID-19 from December 2019 into January 2020.[1] There were 48,588,813 confirmed cases by the beginning of November 2020 and 1,233,212 deaths worldwide.[2] The United States had the largest number of cases and deaths for a single country: 8,346,163 and 224,296, respectively.[2] Unfortunately, included in these numbers are health care professionals. Some observers were astounded by the data because American citizens accounted for only 4 percent of the world's population.[3,4] Many scientists, physicians, and other knowledgeable individuals worried about future effects of the pandemic because of community spread, and although global leaders reported promising news for an effective vaccine, there is no known cure for the disease.[5] Of immediate concern was the effect of the virus on those patients immunocompromised or suffering from other underlying health conditions and the exposure of health care workers. As medical personnel watched patients and colleagues die despite all intervention efforts, the overwhelming feelings of fatigue and despair emerged. In addition to this, moral distress already evident from a preexisting work environment increased as the scarcity of necessary resources became a reality, thereby compromising personal health and threatening medical decision-making. Hundreds of nurses walked off the job due to the stress of being understaffed, while others issued strike notices.[6,7] Before the pandemic, an estimated 17.5 percent of nurses left the profession as a result of moral distress and eventual burnout.[8]

The coupling of the spiritual and the psycho-emotional components of health with terminal physiological issues, despite treatability, is what necessitates palliative care, a care paradigm that offers spiritual, psychological, and physical care to patients with chronic disease and terminal illness, family members included. But for those working on the front lines, especially amid a pandemic, what are the available resources for them in support of their own well-being? Even absent a pandemic, there is clear evidence of moral distress among health care workers. Moral distress occurs when health care professionals are caught in between their personal values and the care plan for patients and/ or institutional policies. As the COVID-19 pandemic has become one among many stress factors for the general public, it seems inevitable that the same would apply to health care workers. I contend, contrarian positions notwithstanding, that the well-being of practitioners is just as important as the well-being of the patients to whom they render care; this includes chaplains. But I purport that hospital chaplains are more prepared due to their training in responding to spiritual and moral distress. Therefore, the integration of spirituality in self-care is a good remedy for mitigating unhealthy outcomes due to emotional stress. One model we can follow is the palliative care model. To this end, the following is important: (1) that health care professionals incorporate spirituality in their self-care plan; (2) that health care systems revisit policies that undermine institutional ethics; and (3) that health care systems remove barriers that foster unhealthy working conditions, thereby limiting high-quality care delivery.

Moral Distress and Health Care

Moral distress in health care settings has been thoroughly researched for decades, going back to the introductory research of Andrew Jameton, where it was then confined to the practice of nursing. At that time, Jameton described moral distress as when a nurse "knows the right thing to do but institutional constraints make it impossible to pursue the right course of action."[9] Physicians, nurses, and other medical staff can experience moral distress. Over the years, the term has found wide application within the health care field. According to Marcia Day Childress, associate professor of medical education at the University of Virginia School of Medicine, moral distress is "poorly understood and rarely discussed." However, while most understand that physicians experience moral distress, the experience of nurses offers the most insight.[10]

Spirituality and Religion in Health Care

Spirituality and religion are often conflated and used synonymously. However, over the years the two terms have become distinctly defined.[11] Spirituality and religion in health care have been studied extensively over the years with the goal of trying to understand how this construct affects patient-physician relationships, patient decision-making, and post-operative recovery, as well as how spirituality and religion are resourced for strength in coping through life's difficult situations.[12,13] As the literature shows, the way in which spirituality may serve as a source of strength for patients may be of benefit to health care providers as well.[14] Dr. Jeannette South-Paul, professor and chair emeritus, family medicine at the University of Pittsburgh School of Medicine, stated the following when asked how she has used her faith in the practice of medicine:

> *"Early in my career I recognized that medicine does not provide answers and cures for everything. But my faith supports me in the knowledge that even when I am running out of traditional medical interventions, my role as a healer has not ended. I can provide emotional and spiritual support, assist the patient in understanding what we know, what is experimental, and where we have limited data but where I am willing to pray with them for the intercession of the Greatest Physician. I assure them that I allow Him to touch my mind and my hands to deliver the best care possible for them."*

Defining Spirituality

Spirituality is the instrument that enables humans to foster the ability to reconcile meaning and purpose amid suffering. As evidenced in scholarly literature, spirituality is broadly defined in relation to religion or religiosity. According to Barry Callen, professor emeritus of Christian studies at Anderson University, spirituality is "trans-religious."[15] Over the previous decades, the definition of spirituality has been expanded. Heelas and Woodhead suggest the growing influence of spirituality in contrast to the declining influence of religion is perhaps the most significant event since the Protestant Reformation of the 16th century.[16] Therefore, it may be possible to assume that the corollary between spirituality's growth and religion's decline is due to this "trans-religious" appeal.

At the Summit on Spirituality by the Association for Spiritual, Ethical, and Religious Values in Counseling in 1995, spirituality was defined as:

> *"the animating force in life, represented by such images as breath, wind, vigor, and courage. Spirituality is the infusion and drawing out of spirit in one's life. It is experienced as an active and passive process. Spirituality also is described as a capacity and tendency that is innate and unique to all persons. This spiritual tendency moves the individual towards knowledge, love, meaning, hope, transcendence, connectedness, and compassion. Spirituality includes one's capacity for creativity, growth, and the development of a values system. Spirituality encompasses the religions, spiritual, and transpersonal."*[17]

Herein we see spirituality identified as a process one participates in as well as a capacity from within.

Differentiating Spirituality and Religion

While these concepts are important within the clinical environment, defining spirituality and religion are difficult. The two terms have often been used interchangeably and often inconsistently despite evolved distinctions in definition.[14,18] In addition, scholars also suggest that the terms spirituality and religion are ambiguously defined.[18,19] There has been increasing interest in spirituality and religion over the last few decades from social scientists[18] and mental health professionals.[20] In agreeing with the distinction that spirituality is broader than religion, Daniel Sulmasy suggests not everyone is religious but all are spiritual, even in the sense that those who may reject the notion of a transcendent being, whether or not they call the transcendent "God," are in relationship with the transcendent by their mere rejection.[14]

The *Handbook of the Psychology of Religion and Spirituality* reports that one in four people in the United States identify as "spiritual but not religious."[19] What Hill and co-authors state, based on a study performed by Sheridan, Bullis, Adcock, Berlin, and Miller, is that fewer than 50 percent of licensed social workers, licensed professional counselors, and psychologists believe that there is a God of transcendence and power. The same study also reports that fewer than 50 percent of clinical and counseling psychologists view religion as very or fairly important to them while over 70 percent note the importance of spirituality.[20] Why this is important is because the majority of those studied accept spirituality in some form. Also, as medical professionals seek ways to cope amid COVID-19, spirituality and peer support can be an important agency.

Building Resilience in Crises and the Importance of Chaplaincy

Palliative care is interdisciplinary in its approach. Many suggest that teamwork is the only way to provide holistic care to the patient.[21] I contend that this same model of teamwork should be examined for resiliency among health care providers. The development of a peer support system can be critical. The role and responsibility of the chaplain should not be overlooked or undervalued in this team approach, especially in mitigating moral or spiritual distress. According to Frances Norwood, the chaplain operates and navigates along the margins within the health care construct, among "competing structures and ideologies."[22] These structures and ideologies must be considered in any remediation effort.

In most clinical settings, it is the hospital chaplain who offers spiritual care. However, literature shows that many benefits chaplains bring to the clinical environment have gone undocumented.[23] Various members of the health care team, including nurses, physicians, and social workers, as well as chaplains, can offer spiritual care.[24] Particularly, Kara Carpenter and co-authors offer four recommendations for nurses who are engaging spirituality in their encounter with patients, three of which are: (1) evaluate your own sense of spirituality; (2) be mindful to nurture your spirituality; and (3) be clear about the meaning and purpose of your roles.[25] Being comfortable in supporting patients can be the first step in the building of resilience.

Professional chaplaincy has changed over the past 50 years from being marginally qualified to requiring professional certifications. The 2005 Comprehensive Accreditation Manual for Hospitals infers that hospital chaplains should be professionally qualified "through certification or applicable licensure."[26] Chaplains are equipped and trained to deal with various moments of crisis, engaging multiple cultures and faith traditions with compassion and sensitivity, while listening for signs of spiritual distress, anger, and fear.[27] Therefore, this same skill can and should officially be made available in supporting the medical team. However, it should be noted that even chaplains have been affected by this pandemic in some way. The Rev. Paul Edwards, director of spiritual care at Jefferson Memorial Hospital in Pittsburgh, shares this reflection:

"The limitations of wearing the appropriate PPE (as required by policy) has impacted the, might I say, 'personal' component in visits that are done. Patients who prefer to see my face, to touch/hold my hands (especially when prayers are being said),

cannot have that interaction. It is as difficult for the patient as it is for me, as the chaplain. My style is very personal and has left me wondering about my ability to genuinely transmit the warmth, compassion, and concern, behind a mask, where no one can see my expressions."

Literature notes that chaplains not only provide spiritual support to patients but are also available to support the medical staff.[26] Mohrmann reminds us that the work of practicing medicine and offering patient care is saturated with spiritual significance not only for the patients but also for the care providers, and it is important that chaplains make sure these moments of spiritual significance are "acknowledged, wrestled with, celebrated, and mourned."[24]

Medical School Education

How are medical students prepared for the stress of the profession? As important as cultural competency is to the delivery of quality care, so too is the corresponding understanding of the spiritual beliefs, practices, and possible effects spirituality can have on patient decision-making, health outcomes, well-being of family members, and for health care professionals. As mentioned earlier, health care professionals should take the opportunity to acknowledge and nurture their own spirituality.

Preparing medical residents and interns for resilience is important as well. In further advocating the palliative care model as an example for building resiliency among practitioners, literature shows there were clearly insufficiencies in medical school curriculum in Germany and the United States several years ago. But in regard to incorporating spirituality within the palliative care curricula, current research seems to indicate medical schools are still lacking in that area. Weissman and co-authors describe a grant program offered to 16 qualifying medical schools over three years with the expressed purpose of developing three important components of palliative care education:

(1) experiential opportunities for students in their final two years of medical school;

(2) an elective experiential opportunity in the final two years; and

(3) a faculty development program to give faculty the foundations in providing and supervising these palliative care experiences.[28]

According to the information provided by the institutions that applied for funding, their concept of experiential learning involved accompanying a hospice nurse on a home visit and attending interdisciplinary team meetings, as well as observing structured clinical encounters. While this form of training is important, the authors describe it as trying to teach a person how to drive while they sit in the back seat and watch.[28] What they consider to be ideal for medical school curricula are:

(1) supervised experiential opportunities where students perform patient palliative care assessments, perform physical exams, and develop care plans based on the assessment;

(2) learning communications skills through supervised practice with feedback;

(3) knowledge transfer of core palliative care principles with hospice and palliative medicine (HPM) certified faculty;

(4) reflective time where the student can process his or her own emotions as a result of caring for terminal and dying patients; and

(5) interdisciplinary participation with hospice and palliative care teams sharing, based on their own assessments and examinations of patients.[28]

They further recommend moving away from observation and simulation-based instruction to more hands-on clinical encounters examining real patients as they struggle physically, psychosocially, and spiritually.[28]

In a similar study of medical students at Harvard-affiliated hospitals without required palliative care rotations, Smith and Schaefer surveyed 88 students in their last four months of the 2012–13 academic year.[29] What they discovered was 26 percent of the students never cared for a patient who died, 55 percent never delivered significantly bad news, and 38 percent never worked with a palliative care clinician. Of the 74 percent of students who cared for a dying patient, 84 percent had one or more patient deaths that were not followed up with a debriefing, and 56 percent of the students who cared for a dying patient were never debriefed.[29] In terms of student evaluations of training, 83 percent of the 88 students who responded to the survey expressed the desire for more education on caring for dying and terminally ill patients. Also, almost 50 percent of the students reported caring for dying patients is depressing, 37 percent reported they would feel guilty if a patient died, and 24 percent stated they would be reticent in facing the emotional distress of family members of a dying patient.[29] This information supports the proposal that spirituality courses in medical school curricula should be more extensive than simply covering the anthropology of religion.

While it is important to understand different faiths and belief systems, what is more important is exploring how physicians process and reflect on their own spirituality when facing the death of others. This is especially relevant amid a pandemic like COVID-19. Reflection techniques used in clinical pastoral education would be a good tool to use in debriefing medical students.

Opportunities to nurture one's own spirituality as well as supporting dying patients who are suffering with understanding existential meaning, purpose, and hope can be addressed outside the medical school curriculum through various workshops or conferences. One such program that was studied by Maria Wasner and co-authors was a three-and-a-half-day training called "Wisdom and Compassion in Care for the Dying," a training based in Buddhist practices designed to help medical professionals and volunteers recognize the different aspects of suffering and reflect on their own fears of death.[30] Those who attended the training completed evaluations afterward. According to their findings, before attending the training, 25 percent of the attendees reported their own emotions were a problem, 31 percent reported difficulty communicating with dying patients and their families, and 27 percent reported discomfort with dealing with difficult family members. After the training, 77 percent reported an improvement in their ability to cope with these difficulties.[30] What is being proposed is the need for the integration of more reflective processing in the training, a technique board-certified chaplains can facilitate. Again, the purpose is to lessen the degree of emotional, psychological, or spiritual distress of the clinician. An example of one school that has incorporated this technique is Massachusetts General Hospital in Boston.

Barriers to Resilience

At a time when hospital administrators are looking for ways to contain costs, many hospital chaplains are concerned that the bull's-eye is on their departments.[31] Also, the role and importance of the hospital chaplain is viewed differently by members of various hospital departments, according to an extensive study by Flannelly et al., a national survey of hospital directors of medicine, nursing, social services, and pastoral care.[21] The survey evaluated seven categories of the chaplain's roles: grief and death, prayer, emotional support, religious services and rituals, consultation and advocacy, community liaison/outreach, and directives and donations. Results of the survey showed that medical directors rated most of these categories lower in importance for chaplains than did any of the other three disciplines. The authors believe this is because physicians view chaplains in limited traditional roles.[21]

There are certainly financial and structural barriers that prevent the full utilization of chaplains. Dr. Harold Koenig recalls how in 1991 the decision was made in Georgia to discontinue the services of full-time chaplains in the state psychiatric hospitals and prisons because of a budget deficit. Some of these chaplains were later replaced with contract chaplains or volunteers.[23] This is still a concern where for-profit corporations are taking over hospitals.[23] Some viewed health care reform as another determinant of how and if chaplains would be utilized in hospitals. In a survey of 370 spiritual care department directors, 27 percent reported that health care reform impacted them either through the downsizing of staff or the elimination of clinical pastoral education (CPE) training.[31] Commenting on how the pandemic has affected the ability to offer pastoral care, the Rev.

Richard Freeman, director of spiritual care at UPMC Children's Hospital in Pittsburgh, stated:

"Spiritual/Pastoral Care practices are significantly dependent on philanthropy. The pandemic has placed enormous strains on development departments' capacity to resource our work."

Norwood argues that chaplains must finesse their way through the structures of hospitals, balancing between embracing religion and distancing themselves from medicine.[22] Managed care policies, the focus on documentation for electronic data records, and cost-cutting measures are at times at odds with what clinicians understand to be the primary focus—patient care, thereby creating ethical dilemmas.[8]

Conclusion

The emotional toll medical professionals face has been exacerbated as a result of the pandemic. Working in the tension of offering the best patient-centered care possible, while risking one's own life in the process due to limited supplies of personal protective equipment even as you watch colleagues die due to exposure, invokes an internal war of fear versus courage. In addition, when the degree of sickness outweighs the ability to treat in accordance with one's values because the resources needed are in limited supply and the decision must be made to terminate treatment, moral distress increases beyond pre-pandemic conditions. To avoid burnout, clinicians need to find a way to build resilience. Their support is already within arm's reach, and it's the chaplain. Using the paradigm in place that has worked with families and loved ones in their deepest moment of pain and grief as one transitions from life as we know it, the medical staff can build a network of peer support with the chaplain as its anchor. Whether clinicians consider themselves religious, spiritual, areligious, or atheist, the chaplain is skilled enough to connect with the moral epicenter of the person. However, to make this possible, perceptions about the role of the chaplain, in addition to institutional policies that have diminished the value of the office, must be reviewed and remedied.

Rev. John C. Welch, PhD
Adjunct Professor of Business Ethics
University of Pittsburgh Katz Graduate School of Business

Endnotes

1. WHO. Timeline of WHO's Response to COVID-19. World Health Organization. https://www.who.int/news-room/detail/29-06-2020-covidtimeline. Published 2020. Accessed August 1, 2020, 2020.

2. Countries Where COVID-19 Has Spread. Woldometer. https://www.worldometers.info/coronavirus/countries-where-coronavirus-has-spread/. Published 2020. Accessed November 1, 2020, 2020.

3. Andrew S. The US Has 4% of the World's Population but 25% of Its Coronavirus Cases. 2020. https://www.cnn.com/2020/06/30/health/us-coronavirus-toll-in-numbers-june-trnd/index.html. Published June 30, 2020. Accessed September 1, 2020.

4. AP. Europe Watches in Alarm as U.S. Tops 5 Million COVID-19 Cases. 2020. https://www.nbcnews.com/health/health-news/europe-watches-alarm-u-s-tops-5-million-covid-19-n1236261. Published August 10, 2020. Accessed August 10, 2020.

5. Zimmer C, Corum J, Wee S-L. Coronavirus Vaccine Tracker. 2020. https://www.nytimes.com/interactive/2020/science/coronavirus-vaccine-tracker.html Published August 31, 2020. Accessed October 1, 2020.

6. Akhtar A. 800 Nurses in Pennsylvania Staged a Walkout Today to Protest Dangerous Working Conditions That They Say are Caused by Understaffing. *Business Insider.* 2020. https://news.yahoo.com/800-nurses-pennsylvania-staged-walkout-221134090.html. Published November 17, 2020. Accessed November 20, 2020.

7. Gartland M. New Rochelle Nurses Vow Strike as COVID Surges. *New York Daily News*. 2020. https://www.msn.com/en-us/health/medical/new-rochelle-nurses-vow-strike-as-covid-surges/ar-BB1bdJ7a. Published November 21, 2020. Accessed November 21, 2020.

8. Rushton CH. Creating a Culture of Ethical Practice in Health Care Delivery Systems. *Nursing, Ethics, and Health Policy, Special Report, Hastings Center Report*. 2016;46(5):S28-31.

9. Jameton A. *Nursing Practice: The Ethical Issues*. Englewood Cliffs, NJ: Pearson College Div.; 1984.

10. Hamric AB, Davis WS, Childress MD. Moral Distress in Healthcare Professionals: What Is It and What Can We Do about It? *The Pharos of Alpha Omega Alpha – Honor Medical Society Alpha Omega Alpha*.69(1):16-23.

11. Pargament KI. The Psychology of Religion and Spirituality? Yes and No. *The International Journal for the Psychology of Religion*. 1999;9(1):3-16.

12. Hebert R, Jenckes M, Ford D, O'Connor D, Cooper L. Patient Perspectives on Spirituality and the Patient-Physician Relationship. *Journal of General Internal Medicine*. 2001;16(10):685-692.

13. Powell L, Shahabi L, Thoresen C. Religion and Spirituality. Linkages to Physical Health. *The American Psychologist*. 2003;58(1):36-52.

14. Sulmasy DP. Is Medicine a Spiritual Practice? *Academic Medicine*. 1999;74(9):1002-1005.

15. Callen BL. *Authentic Spirituality: Moving Beyond Mere Religion*. Lexington, KY: Emeth Press; 2001.

16. Heelas P, Woodhead L. *The Spiritual Revolution: Why Religion is Givng Way to Spirituality*. Malden, MA: Blackwell Publishing; 2005.

17. Smith L. Conceptualizing Spirituality and Religion in Counseling: Where We've Come From, Where We Are, and Where We Are Going. *American Journal of Pastoral Counseling*. 2007;42:4-21.

18. Zinnbauer BJ, Pargament KI, Cole B, et al. Religion and Spirituality: Unfuzzying the Fuzzy. *Journal for the Scientific Study of Religion*. 1997;36(4):549.

19. Oman D. Defining Religion and Spirituality. In: *Handbook of the Psychology of Religion and Spirituality, ed. R. F. Paloutzian & C. L. Park*. 2 ed. New York: Guilford; 2013.

20. Hill PC, Pargament KI, Hood RW, et al. Conceptualizing Religion and Spirituality: Points of Commonality, Points of Departure. *Journal for the Theory of Social Behaviour.* 2000;30(1):51-77.

21. Flannelly KJ, Galek K, Bucchino J, Handzo GF, Tannenbaum HP. Department Directors' Perceptions of the Roles and Functions of Hospital Chaplains: A National Survey. *Hospital Topics.* 2005;83(4):19-28.

22. Norwood F. The Ambivalent Chaplain: Negotiating Structural and Ideological Difference on the Margins of Modern-Day Hospital Medicine. *Medical Anthropology.* 2006;25(1):1-29.

23. Koenig HG. Why Research is Important for Chaplains. *Journal of Health Care Chaplaincy.* 2008;14(2):83-90.

24. Mohrmann ME. Ethical Grounding for a Profession of Hospital Chaplaincy. 2008.

25. Carpenter K, Girvin L, Kitner W, Ruth-Sahd LA. Spirituality: A Dimension of Holistic Critical Care Nursing. *Dimensions of Critical Care Nursing.* 2008;27(1):16-20.

26. McClung E, Grossoehme D, Jacobson A. Collaborating with Chaplains to Meet Spiritual Needs. *MEDSURG Nursing: Official Journal of the Academy of Medical-Surgical Nurses.* 2006;15(3):147-156.

27. Snorton TE. Setting Common Standards for Professional Chaplains in an Age of Diversity. *Southern Medical Journal.* 2006;99(6):660-662.

28. Weissman DE, Quill TE, Block SD. Missed Opportunities in Medical Student Education. *Journal of Palliative Medicine.* 2010;13(5):489-490.

29. Smith GM, Schaefer KG. Missed Opportunities To Train Medical Students in Generalist Palliative Care during Core Clerkships. *Journal of Palliative Medicine.* 2014;17(12):1344-1347.

30. Wasner M, Longaker C, Fegg M, Borasio G. Effects of Spiritual Care Training for Palliative Care Professionals. *Palliative Medicine.* 2005;19(2):99-104.

31. VandeCreek L. How Has Health Care Reform Affected Professional Chaplaincy Programs and How Are Department Directors Responding? *Journal of Health Care Chaplaincy.* 2000;10(1):7-17.

ACKNOWLEDGMENTS

We want to thank the hundreds of thousands of doctors who go to hospitals and clinics every day, arriving early, staying late, taking calls through dark hours and long weekends to care for us, our families, our friends, and our communities. Thank you for your knowledge, skills, dedication, and for caring for us, whether young or old, rich or poor, conscious or not—all of us, with our illnesses and injuries. This book is about caring for you, about your health and wellbeing, and about how we can come together to support you when you find yourself worn out, up against a wall, stressed, fatigued, or burned out.

We owe a debt of gratitude to the author contributors to this book, including doctors, coaches, counselors, spiritual caregivers, and others, who have shared their knowledge, wisdom, experiences, and stories. We appreciate your commitment to caring for those who care for us—our physicians.

We are grateful to Janet Griffin, who spent untold hours carefully copyediting each chapter, page by page, line by line, cleaning up typos, correcting grammar, and re-arranging our sometimes-awkward phrasing. We are indebted to Teri Mulvey for professionally and patiently assuring the accuracy and consistency of our bibliographies and references.

We want to give special thanks to our peer reviewers: Jeffrey Kuhlman, Jessica Baird-Wertman, Theresa Herbert, Eric Shadle, Loice Swisher, Cindy Boskind, and Roger Woodruff. They provided important suggestions about our manuscript to make it even more compelling. We appreciate the time, energy, and expertise they contributed.

We could never have completed this work without the support, professionalism, courtesy, and counsel of the staff at AdventHealth Press, including Denise Putt, Caryn McCleskey, Todd Chobotar, and the rest of their team—Lillian Boyd, Sheila Draper, and Danica Eylenstein. Thank you for encouraging us, guiding us, and helping us bring this book to life.

ABOUT THE EDITORS

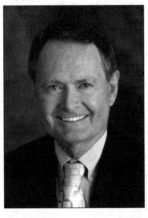

Ted Hamilton, MD, MBA, is chief mission integration officer for AdventHealth. He provides direction and oversight of mission and ministry, developing and implementing strategy and incorporating mission across all the organization's inpatient and outpatient areas. A graduate of the Loma Linda University School of Medicine, Hamilton completed his family practice training at Florida Hospital. He also earned a master's degree in business administration. He is co-editor of *Transforming the Heart of Practice: An Organizational and Personal Approach to Physician Well-being,* published in 2019.

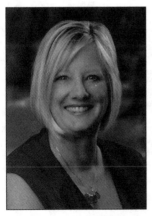

Dianne McCallister, MD, MBA, a board-certified internist and former chief medical officer, has extensive administrative and quality improvement experience. Dianne is co-founder of the Coalition for Physician Well-Being and co-editor of the book *Transforming the Heart of Practice: An Organizational and Personal Approach to Physician Wellbeing* (Springer 2019). She is a published author, with book chapters on quality, patient safety, and EMCO program development.

Dr. McCallister speaks nationally and internationally on physician well-being and other topics.

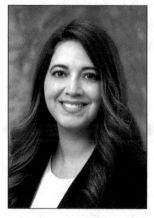

DeAnna Santana-Cebollero, PhD, is the director of physician well-being and engagement for AdventHealth. In her current role, she focuses on the development of mission-specific initiatives, such as the development of a mission fit selection tool, as well as onboarding, mentor, and integration programs to increase the well-being and engagement of physicians and advanced practice providers. DeAnna graduated from Walden University with her PhD in industrial-organizational psychology, where she focused her research on physician well-being.

ABOUT THE AUTHORS

Bryant Adibe, MD, serves as system vice president and chief wellness officer for the Rush University System for Health in Chicago, Illinois. He holds the distinction of off-site, full professor of organizational change and leadership at the University of Southern California and visiting professor of health policy at Guangzhou Medical University in Guangzhou, China. Dr. Adibe earned his medical degree from the University of Florida College of Medicine and studied health policy research and evidence-based health care at Oxford University.

Tania Aylmer, LMHC, is a licensed mental health counselor and received her master's degree in mental health counseling from the University of Central Florida. She currently serves as the clinical professionalism manager for the department of professionalism at AdventHealth. During the peak of COVID-19, she completed mental health well-being rounds to frontline workers and saw firsthand the challenges and emotional distress team members were experiencing. Tania has also developed and offers supportive strategies and interventions to physicians who are demonstrating inappropriate or disruptive behavior.

Burt Bertram, EdD, LMHC, is a Florida-licensed mental health counselor and marriage and family therapist, professor, and author. He has been in private practice in Orlando for over 40 years. His professional counseling is primarily focused on the resolution of sensitive and complex relationship issues in every aspect of life—personal, workplace, and community. For more than a decade, Dr. Bertram was a consulting psychotherapist to the Center for Physician Well-Being (AdventHealth/ Florida Hospital), where he provided counseling, coaching, and professional development experiences to physicians and advanced practice professionals.

Keith Carter, BSc, MD, FRCPC, is an anesthesiologist/critical care physician, currently practicing at Royal Inland Hospital in Kamloops, British Columbia. He completed his medical training and residency in anesthesia at the University of Calgary, in Calgary, Alberta, and did additional training in trauma/critical care, including an elective at Loma Linda University. Regarding the context of his contribution to the book, he served as head of anesthesia and in charge of the "COVID Airway Response Team" at the time of its writing.

Jessica ChenFeng, PhD, LMFT, is associate professor of medical education and associate director of physician vitality at Loma Linda University Health. She is an alumna of UCLA, Fuller Theological Seminary, and Loma Linda University. Growing up in Los Angeles in a Taiwanese immigrant family and in the Asian American Christian church has shaped her research, teaching, and clinical work around sociocontextual issues such as gender, race, generation, and spirituality.

Calvin Chou, MD, PhD, is professor of clinical medicine at the University of California at San Francisco and staff physician at the Veterans Affairs Health Care System in San Francisco. As senior faculty advisor for external education with the Academy of Communication in Healthcare (ACH), he is recognized internationally for leading workshops in relationship-centered communication, feedback, conflict, and remediation in health professions education. He is co-editor of the books *Remediation in Medical Education: A Midcourse Correction* and *Communication Rx: Transforming Healthcare Through Relationship-Centered Communication.*

Gregory K. Ellis, MDiv, BCC, serves as executive director of mission and ministry for AdventHealth Central Florida Division. Greg earned his master of divinity degree from Andrews University and is a board-certified chaplain with the Association of Professional Chaplains. He is an ordained Seventh-day Adventist minister and endorsed by Adventist Chaplaincy Ministries. One of his areas of passion is the integration of spiritual care within the health care environment, aligning the mind, body, and spirit.

Liz Ferron, MSW, LICSW, is a licensed independent clinical social worker and has served as the physician practice lead for VITAL WorkLife since 2001. Liz received her master's degree in social work from the University of Minnesota in Minneapolis, Minnesota. Liz has contributed to the development and analysis of VITAL WorkLife's national surveys, has presented on physician well-being at national and regional conferences, and has been published in several medical journals. Currently, Liz provides training and consultation to health care administrators and individual practitioners in the areas of stress management, navigating change, and effective communication.

Kathy Gibney, PhD, LP, ABPP, is a diplomate of the American Board of Professional Psychology with 37 years of experience in counseling, consulting, education, and training to individuals, families, groups, organizations, and communities. She received her doctoral training in psychology at Northeastern University and her clinical training at BU Medical Center and the Center for Multicultural Psychology. She is certified in Critical Incident Debriefing. Kathy has worked in a variety of clinical settings and has taught at universities, including the University of Notre Dame where she was awarded the Kaneb teaching award. Her past experiences have increased her passion and appreciation for the personal and professional journeys that can change people's hearts.

Pam Guler, MHA, FACHE, serves as vice president and chief experience officer for AdventHealth. She holds a master of healthcare administration from the University of South Florida. She leads efforts across AdventHealth focused on ensuring an exceptional experience for patients, families, and all consumers, placing particular emphasis on the culture and service standards of the organization with evidence-based methods of communication between clinicians and patients as one of the key drivers of experience and ultimate outcomes.

Tyon Hall, PhD, graduated from Florida State University with a bachelor's degree in psychology and double-minored in sociology and African American studies. She has a master's and holds a doctorate degree from Nova Southeastern University with a specialization in marriage and family therapy. Dr. Hall is an experienced adjunct professor and researcher. She is a published author and presenter on topics related to trauma, crisis management, and therapy. She has been featured on podcasts related to healing racial trauma and believes in the importance of providing a safe, culturally competent, whole-person approach in the treatment of therapy to health care providers.

Malcolm Herring, MD, served for 32 years as a practicing vascular surgeon and for ten years in the Coalition for Physician Well-Being. He has worked with physicians and their spouses on issues of spiritual formation, well-being, engagement, and mission alignment, and teaches life-centered mentoring for physicians. His book, *The Physician Champion*, was written to help physician leaders with those issues.

Juleun A. Johnson, DMin, serves as director of mission and ministry for AdventHealth in Central Florida. He also serves as lead chaplain at AdventHealth Celebration. He holds a doctor of ministry from the Claremont School of Theology. His dissertation focused on end-of-life care and education for clergy and community. He is the author of two books: *Five Minutes On Purpose* and *The Built to Thrive Discovery Guide*. He has written articles for international journals and publications. He has served as an adjunct professor at AdventHealth University and Gulf Coast State College and as doctoral advisor at Denver Seminary. His research interests include grief, gratitude, and resilience.

Rachel Forbes Kaufman, a credentialed spiritual companion, writes and teaches about the intersection of spirituality and physician well-being. She is the founding director of the Medical Professionals Retirement Institute, and her practice is dedicated to helping medical professionals transcend into a purpose-filled second half of life.

Hobart Lee, MD, FAAFP, is an associate professor at the Loma Linda University Medical School and the LLUHEC Family Medicine Residency program director. He completed medical school at the Perelman School of Medicine at the University of Pennsylvania, and his family medicine residency and Academic

Faculty Development Fellowship at the University of Michigan. He is passionate about leadership development and the connection between faith, spirituality, and medicine.

Katherine Lundrigan, MBA, CTAGME, is currently an associate program director of the Loma Linda University Family Medicine Residency program. She has worked in graduate medical education for over a decade and enjoys creating systems that encourage medical professionals at every stage of their careers to learn and grow.

Omayra Mansfield, MD, MHA, FACEP, is a board-certified emergency medicine physician. She is the vice president and chief medical officer at AdventHealth Apopka and AdventHealth Winter Garden. She obtained her medical degree and master of healthcare administration at the University of Florida and completed her residency at Carolinas Medical Center. She is a fellow with the American College of Emergency Physicians. Dr. Mansfield co-authored The Trust Transformation, a workshop that helps participants transform and improve the relationships in their lives by building a foundation of trust. Her primary areas of interest are improving the physician and patient experience.

Reina Mayor, MD, completed her undergraduate degree in biology at San Diego State University. She attended George Washington University School of Medicine. She completed her pediatric residency at Texas Children's Hospital and neonatology fellowship at University of Texas Southwestern. Dr. Mayor has practiced neonatology at AdventHealth for six years. Her interests focus on postpartum depression and maternal anxiety in NICU moms.

Carla Park, PhD, is the executive director for faith community strategy at the corporate office of AdventHealth and assistant to the president for mission at AdventHealth University. Before coming to AdventHealth, she worked as the assistant vice president for mission at Loma Linda University Health, was the director of a center for whole-person care at Loma Linda University, and taught as a university professor of religion and medicine. In 2015, she was lead producer of the award-winning film *A Certain Kind of Light*, a short-form documentary film on whole-person care. She has degrees in the fields of nursing (RN), marriage and family counseling (MS), public health education (MPH), and a PhD in religious studies from Emory University.

Orlando Jay Perez, MDiv, ACPE-certified educator and vice president of mission and ministry, is responsible for the integration of mission across AdventHealth, chaplaincy services, and mission onboarding for employees and leaders within the company. He previously served as vice president of mission and ministry for the Florida Division. He earned a master's degree in divinity from Andrews University Theological Seminary. Jay is a member of the Association for Clinical Pastoral Education. The passion for reflection and journaling is at the center of his personal formation as a clinical pastoral educator.

Craig Pirner is a managing director at The Advisory Board, a health care research firm, where he leads the leadership development practice. In his 15+ years with the company, Craig has consulted with 200+ health care institutions in the United States, United Kingdom, Australia, and Canada on the design and delivery of leadership development programs. An in-demand keynote speaker, he has facilitated 1,000+ leadership development experiences for clinical and administrative leaders.

Craig graduated summa cum laude from Washington University in St. Louis with a BA in music, political science, and educational studies.

Ramona Reynolds, MDiv, MHA, is an APC Board Certified Chaplain and ACPE Certified Educator at AdventHealth Orlando. She is a graduate of the University of Kentucky, Southern Baptist Theological Seminary, and AdventHealth University. Ramona is married with a teenage son.

Robert Rodgers, MD, is a family physician with over 25 years of experience, the last 21 of which have been with AdventHealth. He recently accepted a position as the chief medical officer of AdventHealth Senior Care, a new business unit focusing on full-risk clinics for those 65 and older. He received his MD degree from Loma Linda University and then completed his residency training at what was then the Florida Hospital Orlando Family Medicine program. Dr. Rodgers has been married to his wife, Cindy, for 33 years, and they are blessed to have two adult children, Austin and Kelina, and added Victoria as a daughter-in-law just prior to the pandemic shutdown.

Sy Saliba, PhD, serves as director of AdventHealth Leadership Institute with focus on physician and executive leadership development. Previously, as senior vice president for marketing for AdventHealth Central Florida Division, Dr. Saliba was active in the local and the larger global community serving as a board member of the American Heart Association and Orlando Chamber of Commerce.

Martin Schreiber, EdD, is the vice president for the Mission Leadership Institute at Providence St. Joseph Health. Martin has over 20 years of experience working with leaders in architecting and developing culture in the fields of health care, education, and community services. He holds a doctor of education from Loyola University and master's degrees of divinity and applied philosophy. He is the host of the *Healing Stories Podcast* that explores how we integrate our stories to find healing in our lives. Martin grew up in Cleveland, Ohio, and now lives in San Clemente, California, with his wife, Allie, and their four children.

Herbert A. Schumm, MD, FAAFP, is a family physician by training and an administrator by experience. After ten years of private practice, he served as a VPMA and then a medical group president in Lima, OH. In 2016, Herb transitioned to a system role, leading provider professional development with a focus on physician well-being and learning with Mercy Health (now Bon Secours Mercy Health). Herb currently serves as chair of the Huntington University Board of Trustees. He enjoys woodworking, building folk instruments, and investing in the next generation of leaders.

Jocelyn Shaw, MDiv, serves as the senior chaplain for AdventHealth for Children. She has a passion for working in the areas of health care and spirituality. Jocelyn attended Southern Adventist University, receiving a bachelor of arts in pastoral care, followed by completion of her chaplaincy residency in 2012. She attended Andrews University Theological Seminary, completing her master of divinity degree alongside her husband, Martin Shaw. Providing psychosocial emotional and spiritual support to patients, families, and staff members are top priority for Jocelyn.

Jennifer Stanley, MD, is a family physician practicing with Ascension Medical Group in rural Indiana. Having joined Ascension in 2001, she is active in leadership and currently serves as the chair of the AMG Clinician Engagement and Well-Being Council. She also supervises the Life Centered Mentoring Program, which uses a pastoral care approach to support physicians new to the organization. Jennifer recognizes the importance of system response to physician burnout and is active in engaging organizational leadership and physician colleagues in the work to improve clinician experience. Outside her practice, she is a wife and mother of three children.

Rev. John C. Welch, PhD, is a native of Pittsburgh, an ordained minister and bioethicist. He earned his PhD in health care ethics specializing in palliative care. Dr. Welch is an adjunct professor of business ethics at the University of Pittsburgh Katz Graduate School of Business and the University of Pittsburgh's Consortium Ethics Program. Presently, Dr. Welch serves on the Ethics Committee for Forbes Hospital of the Allegheny Health Network and has lectured on numerous subjects, including but not limited to: "Moral Distress," "Christian, Islamic, & Buddhist Perspectives and Medical Decision Making," "African American Perspectives on End of Life," "The Role and Impact of Spirituality in Medicine" and "Implicit Bias and the Ethics of Care."

Mary Wolf, MS, LPC-MH, is the program director for the Avera Medical Group LIGHT Program, a well-being program for physicians, nurse practitioners, and physician assistants. She leads a well-being culture and provides executive coaching for professionals and executives. Mary earned a master's degree in counseling and human resource development and is a licensed professional counselor–mental health and a board-certified coach. Mary is the president of Veritee Partners, a coaching and consulting business that helps physicians, providers, and executives to reduce overwhelm, gain clarity, and create a strategy for better health, relationships, and fulfillment.

J. Michael Yurso, MD, FACS, serves as the vice president of evidence-based practice for AdventHealth. Prior to joining AdventHealth, he practiced the specialty of general surgery at what was then known as Florida Hospital. During this time, he co-founded the Finding Meaning in Medicine® program where he had the opportunity to demonstrate to other physicians and administrators the depth of his listening skills, empathy, compassion, and his ability to invite heartfelt discussion among his physician peers. In his current role, he has the opportunity to combine his experience as a practicing physician and physician leader with the challenges of medical scholarship and team leadership.

ABOUT THE PUBLISHER

AdventHealth is a connected network of care that promotes hope and healing through individualized care that touches the body, mind and spirit to help you feel whole. Our hospitals and care sites across the country are united by one mission: Extending the Healing Ministry of Christ. This faith-based mission guides our skilled and compassionate caregivers to provide expert care that leads the nation in quality, safety, and patient satisfaction.

Over 5 million people visit AdventHealth each year at our award-winning hospitals, physician practices, outpatient clinics, skilled nursing facilities, home health agencies and hospice centers to experience wholistic care for any stage of life and health.

AdventHealth Press publishes content rooted in wholistic health principles to help you feel whole through a variety of physical, emotional, and spiritual wellness resources.

To learn more visit AdventHealthPress.com.

RECOGNITIONS

CLINICAL EXCELLENCE. AdventHealth hospital campuses have been recognized in the top five percent of hospitals in the nation for clinical excellence by Healthgrades. We believe that spiritual and emotional care, along with high-quality clinical care, combine to create the best outcome for our patients.

TOP SAFETY RATINGS. We care for you like we would care for our own loved ones – with compassion and a priority of safety. AdventHealth's hospitals have received grade "A" safety ratings from The Leapfrog Group, the only national rating agency that evaluates how well hospitals protect patients from medical errors, infections, accidents, and injuries.

SPECIALIZED CARE. For over ten years, AdventHealth hospitals have been recognized by U.S. News & World Report as "One of America's Best Hospitals" for clinical specialties such as: Cardiology and Heart Surgery, Orthopedics, Neurology and Neuroscience, Urology, Gynecology, Gastroenterology and GI Surgery, Diabetes and Endocrinology, Pulmonology, Nephrology, and Geriatrics.

AWARD-WINNING TEAM CULTURE. Becker's Hospital Review has recognized AdventHealth as a Top Place to Work in Healthcare based on diversity, team engagement and professional growth. AdventHealth has also been awarded for fostering an engaged workforce, meaning our teams are equipped and empowered in their work as they provide skilled and compassionate care.

WIRED FOR THE FUTURE. The American Hospital Association recognized AdventHealth as a "Most Wired" health system for using the latest technology and innovations to provide cutting-edge, connected care.

PARTNERSHIPS

WALT DISNEY WORLD. AdventHealth has partnered with the Walt Disney World® Resort for over 25 years. As the Official Medical Provider for runDisney and Official Athletic Training Team of ESPN Wide World of Sports, AdventHealth has played a critical role in enhancing the Disney Parks and Resort operations and experiences for athletes.

In 2011, AdventHealth and Disney opened the Walt Disney Pavilion at AdventHealth for Children, which is now one of the premier children's hospitals in the nation, setting standards for innovation, quality and comprehensive care. The child-centric healing environment is designed to keep kids comfortable is complemented by a staff of world-class doctors, specialists, nurses and healthcare professionals utilizing advanced technologies, therapies and treatments. AdventHealth also collaborated with Disney to create AdventHealth Celebration, a cutting-edge comprehensive health facility that was named the "Hospital of the Future" by the *Wall Street Journal*.

STRATEGIC SPORTS. AdventHealth's commitment to whole-athlete care and innovative care models extends throughout our strategic sports partnerships, which span across multiple professional sports leagues including NBA, NFL, NHL, and NASCAR. AdventHealth is the Official Health Care Provider of the Orlando Magic, Lakeland Magic, Orlando Solar Bears, and Sebring International Raceway, Exclusive Hospital of the Tampa Bay Buccaneers, Official Health and Wellness Partner of the Tampa Bay Lightning, as well as the Official Health Care Partner and a Founding Partner of the iconic Daytona International Speedway.

In addition, through our 20+ year partnership with Florida Citrus Sports, AdventHealth has provided comprehensive health care services to collegiate athletes as the Official Health Care Provider for the Cheez-It Bowl and Vrbo Citrus Bowl.

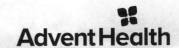

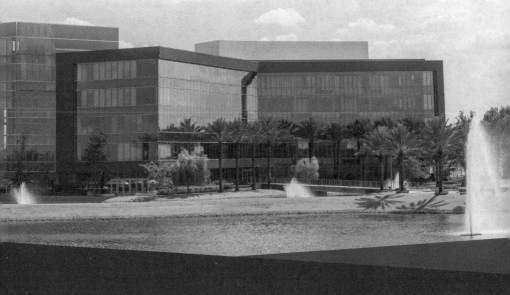

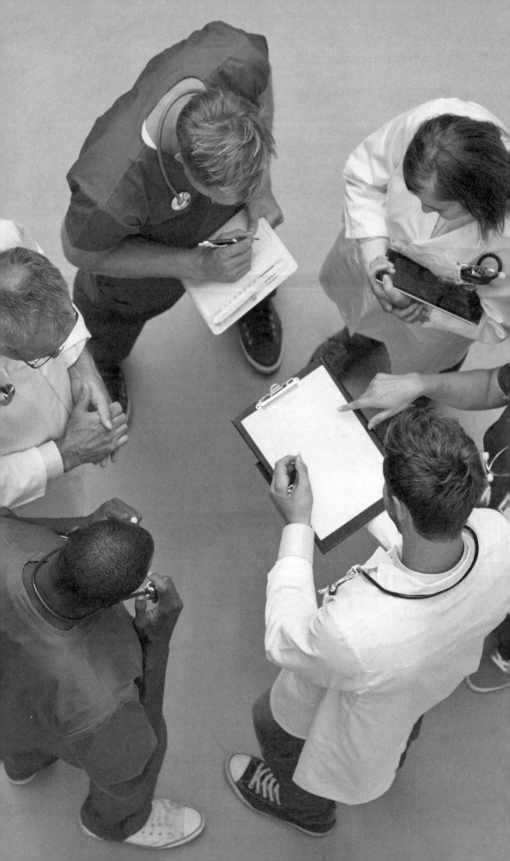

About the Coalition

Wellness Begins Within

Physician well-being and engagement is essential to all mission-focused health care organizations. The Coalition for Physician Well-Being is committed to creating a wholistic paradigm that attends to personal and professional factors that contribute to burnout. By attending to the whole person (body, mind, and spirit) and the professional environment (collegial relationships, workplace environment, and resources for physician well-being), this model advances physician resiliency, sustains families, and promotes a healing culture that will benefit patient care as well as the wellness of the communities we serve.

Find out more at *ForPhysicianWellBeing.org*

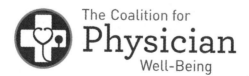

The Coalition for
Physician
Well-Being

INDEX

A

Academy of Communication in Healthcare 138

Accreditation Council of Graduate Medical Education (ACGME) 121, 122, 123, 124, 128, 132

Administrators x, 21, 79, 100, 104, 110, 111, 112, 168, 174, 184, 212, 278

AdventHealth iv, vii, 13, 24, 51, 53, 55, 57, 67, 80, 85, 88, 92, 97, 99, 101, 107, 108, 136, 143, 145, 151, 156, 157, 169, 185, 187, 198, 231, 251, 254, 256, 257, 258, 260, 261, 262, 263, 264, 265, 284

AdventHealth Sebring 185, 187

Adversity 9, 238

Alcohol 10, 48

Anxiety viii, xiii, 5, 6, 19, 23, 28, 29, 36, 48, 50, 58, 61, 82, 98, 102, 105, 106, 122, 154, 181, 204, 206, 230, 252, 253

Authentic/authenticity 148, 155, 281

B

Battle buddy 8, 9, 63

Belonging 104, 238

Bereavement 61

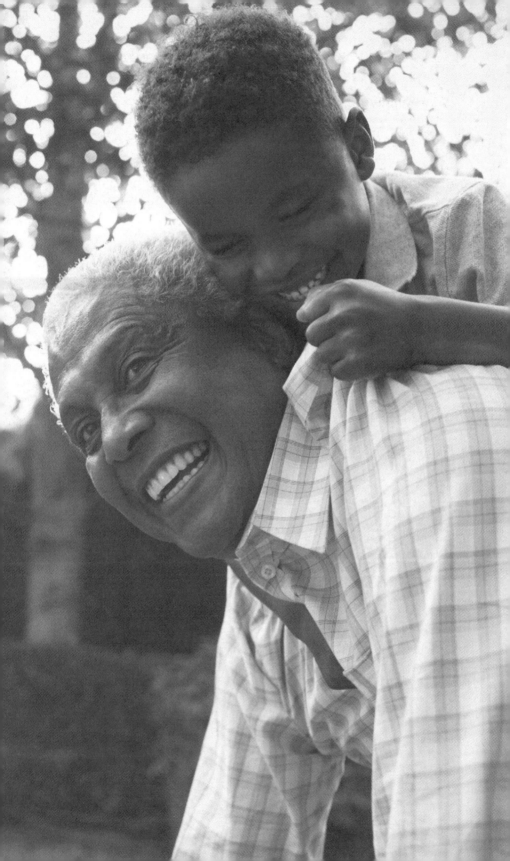

Your Generosity Heals

Generosity is powerful medicine. Studies show that when you give, it reduces stress, alleviates depression, and gives a greater sense of happiness to the giver. It may even lower your blood pressure and extend your life! *

When you give to **AdventHealth's Whole Person Health Education Fund**, you not only help yourself—you help create vital, innovative materials to educate and empower others. You help them discover the healthiest lifestyle on earth. A lifestyle that research shows will add years of health to the lives of those who embrace it.

100 percent of your gift will support these life-changing health resources. To learn more, or to make your Generosity Heals donation today, visit:

www.GenerosityHeals.Health

See website for citations.

LIVE LIFE TO THE FULLEST

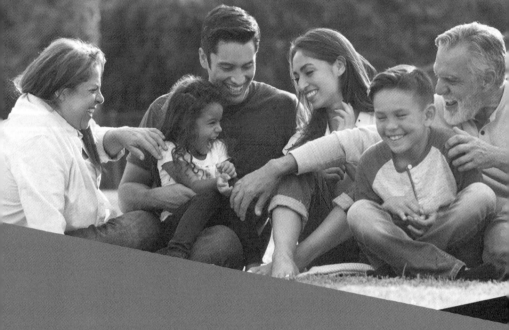

CREATION Life is a faith-based wellness plan for those who want to live healthier and happier lives and share this unique, whole-person health philosophy. By consistently practicing the principles of CREATION Life, we fulfill God's original plan for our lives, which is to live and be happy!

Our mission is to help you live life to the fullest, but we don't stop there. Feeling great is a feeling worth sharing, and we have the tools and resources to equip you for a health ministry.

Visit us at **CREATIONLife.com**
to get started on your journey to feeling whole!

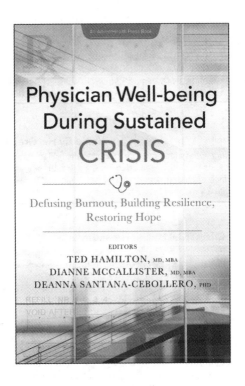

Physician Well-being
During Sustained
CRISIS

Defusing Burnout, Building Resilience,
Restoring Hope

EDITORS
TED HAMILTON, MD, MBA
DIANNE MCCALLISTER, MD, MBA
DEANNA SANTANA-CEBOLLERO, PHD

REGISTER THIS NEW BOOK

Visit AdventHealthPress.com

Benefits of Registering:

FREE **replacement** of lost or damaged book

FREE **audiobook** – *CREATION Life Discovery*

FREE information about new titles and **giveaways**

ADDITIONAL RESOURCES

Transformative Health Care

What if every patient received the kind of focused personal attention Dr. Kuhlman used with three U.S. Presidents? Kuhlman and Peach show how this level of care can be achieved now.

Whole By His Grace

Whole by His Grace was written by women sharing the real struggles, triumphs, and lessons they have learned to inspire you with hope and courage as you face each day. Start each day with a story of hope or finish your day with a sense of His wholeness.

CREATION Health Breakthrough

Blending science and lifestyle recommendations, Monica Reed, MD, prescribes eight essentials that will help reverse harmful health habits and prevent disease. Discover how intentional choices, rest, environment, activity, trust, relationships, outlook, and nutrition can put a person on the road to wellness.

Pain Free For Life

In *Pain Free For Life,* Scott C. Brady, MD, — founder of Florida Hospital's Brady Institute for Health — leads pain-racked readers to a pain-free life using powerful mind-body-spirit strategies — where more than 80 percent of his chronic-pain patients have achieved 80–100 percent pain relief within weeks.

Scalpel Moments

A scalpel moment can be one of painful awareness, disturbing clarity, sorrowful regret. It can also be a moment of positive awakening that can reveal, restore, and renew. Ordained minister Dr. Reaves highlights stories about life's difficult or revealing moments that remove layers of confusion, bitterness, or fear and restore one's trust in God.

The Love Fight

Are you going to fight for love or against each other? The authors illustrate how this common encounter can create a mutually satisfying relationship. Their expertise will walk you through the scrimmage between those who want to accomplish and those who want to relate.

ADDITIONAL RESOURCES

The Hidden Power of Relentless Stewardship

Dr. Jernigan shows how an organization's culture can be molded to create high performance at every level, fulfilling mission and vision, while wisely utilizing - or stewarding - the limited resources of time, money, and energy.

Leadership in the Crucible of Work

What is the first and most important work of a leader? (The answer may surprise you.) In *Leadership in the Crucible of Work*, noted speaker, poet, and college president Dr. Sandy Shugart takes readers on an unforgettable journey to the heart of what it means to become an authentic leader.

Growing Physician Leaders

Retired Army Lieutenant General Mark Hertling applies his four decades of military leadership to the work of healthcare, resulting in a profoundly constructive and practical book with the power to reshape and re-energize any healthcare organization in America today.

Bible Promises to Feel Whole

The Bible is packed with promises on health and healing - from aging to nutrition to rest, from grief to anger to stress. The *Bible Promises to Feel Whole* book collects over 600 scriptures in more than thirty different translations in a convenient pocket size on these topics and more including the CREATION Life principles.

SuperSized Kids

In *SuperSized Kids: How to Rescue Your Child from The Obesity Threat,* Walt Larimore, MD, and Sherri Flynt, MPH, RD, LD, explains step by step, how parents can work to avert the coming childhood obesity crisis by taking control of the weight challenges facing every member of their family.

Simply Healthy: The Art of Eating Well – Diabetes Edition

Simple, enticing, delectable, the recipes in *Simply Healthy: The Art of Eating Well – Diabetes Edition* will convince even the most skeptical that your food can taste good AND be good for you!

AdventHealthPress.com

ADDITIONAL RESOURCES

Life Is Amazing Live It Well

At its heart, Linda's captivating account chronicles the struggle to reconcile her three dreams of experiencing life as a "normal woman" with the tough realities of her medical condition. Her journey is punctuated with insights that are at times humorous, painful, provocative, and life-affirming.

Forgive To Live

In *Forgive To Live: How Forgiveness Can Save Your Life,* Dr. Tibbits presents the scientifically proven steps for forgiveness — taken from the first clinical study of its kind conducted by Stanford University and Florida Hospital.

Forgive To Live Devotional

In his powerful new devotional Dr. Dick Tibbits reveals the secret to forgiveness. This compassionate devotional is a stirring look at the true meaning of forgiveness. Each of the 56 spiritual insights includes motivational Scripture, an inspirational prayer, and two thought-provoking questions. The insights are designed to encourage your journey as you begin to *Forgive to Live.*

Eat Plants, Feel Whole

For over thirty years, Dr. Guthrie has been helping his patients gain better health through an evidence-based, whole-food, plant-based lifestyle. Now, in *Eat Plants, Feel Whole,* he shares not only his years of expertise with you, but the scientific evidence to back it up as well.

Eat Plants Feel Whole Journal

Everything you need to succeed with the *18-day Eat Plants Feel Whole* Plan. The companion journal is an important and welcome addition to the field of healthy nutrition and lifestyle medicine.

AdventHealthPress.com